Dry Eye Syndrome - Modern Diagnostic Techniques and Advanced Treatments

Edited by Felicia M. Ferreri

Published in London, United Kingdom

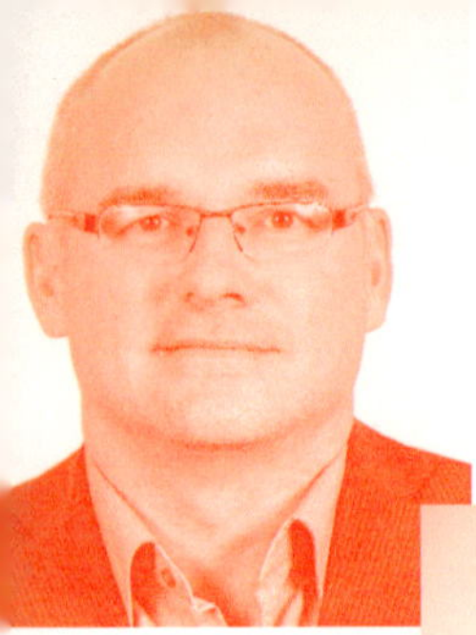
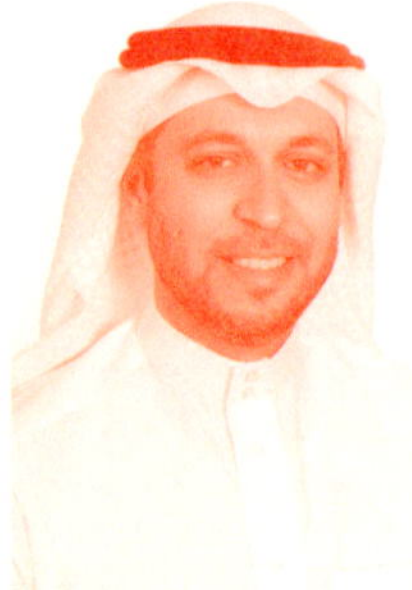
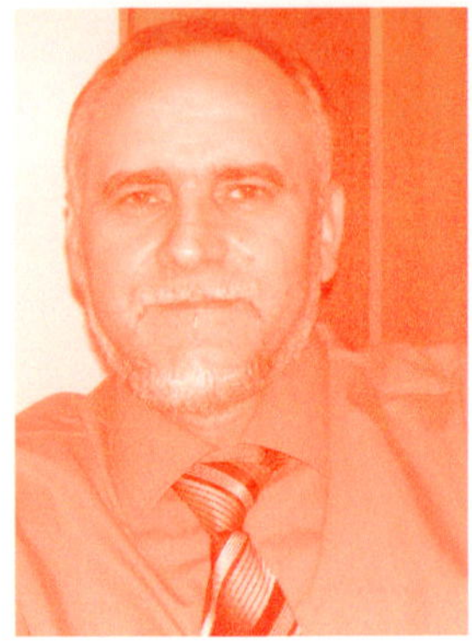
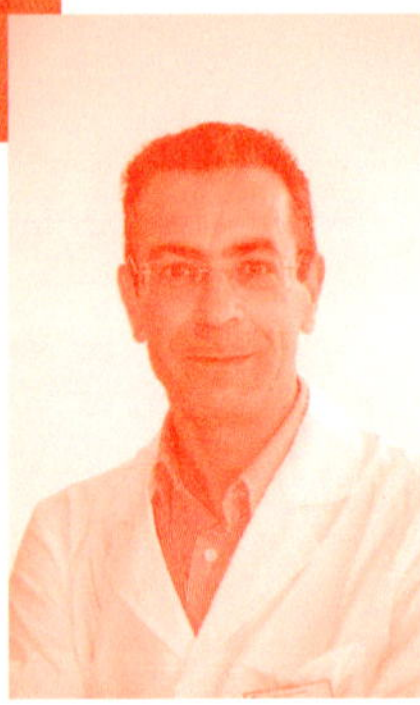
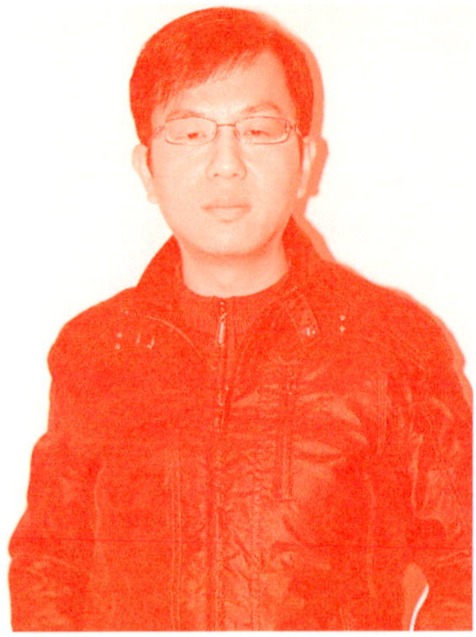
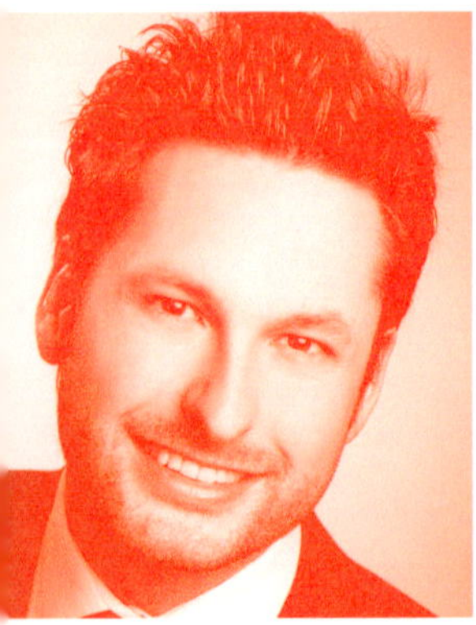
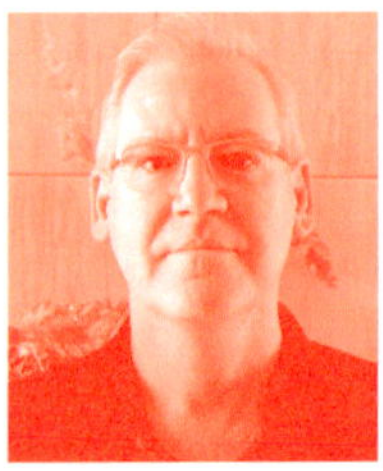

IntechOpen

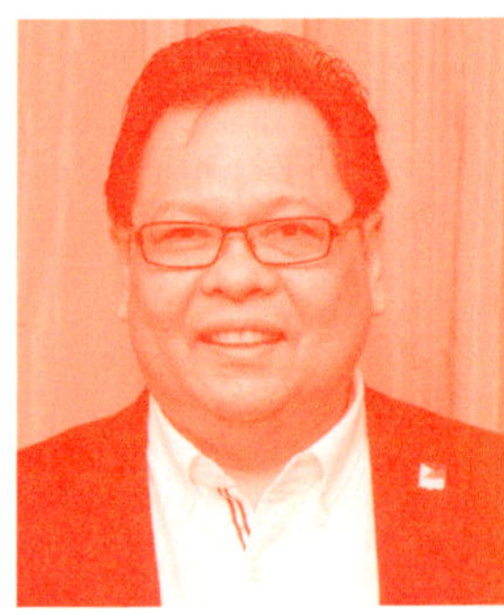
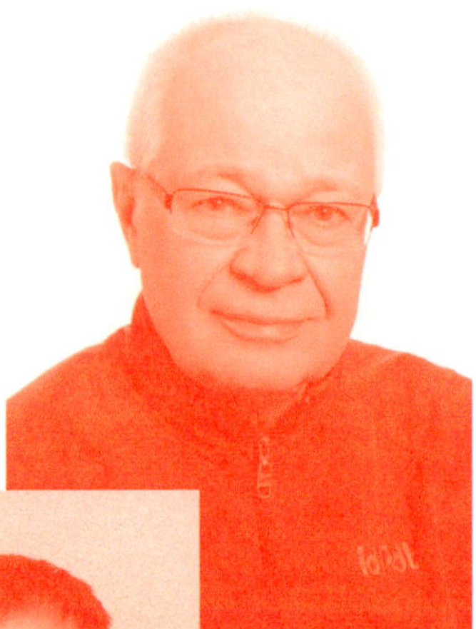
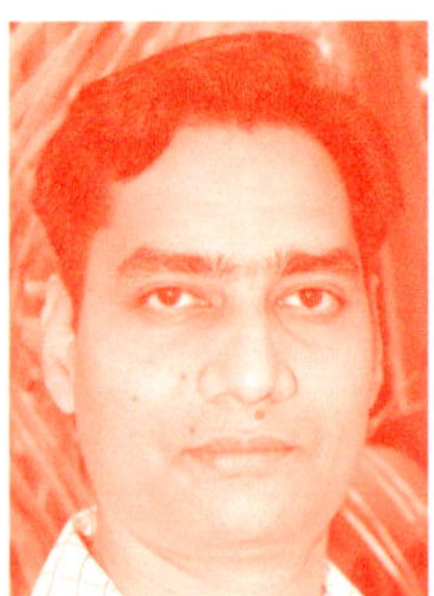
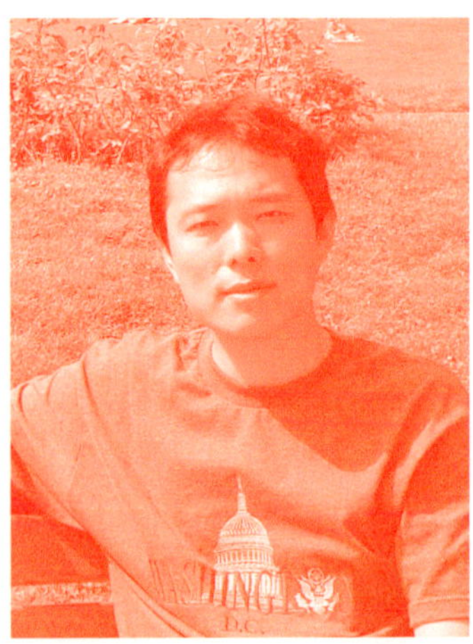
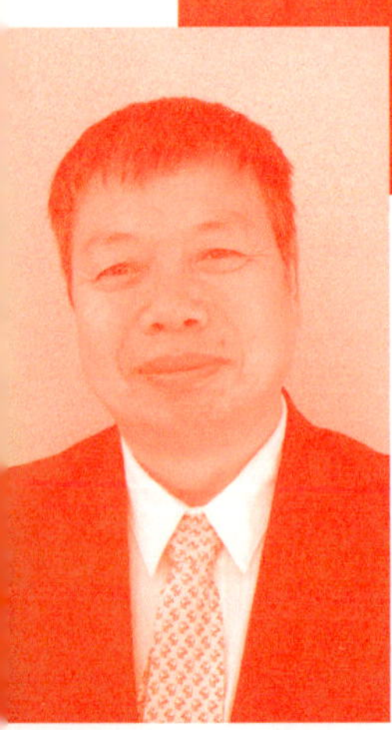
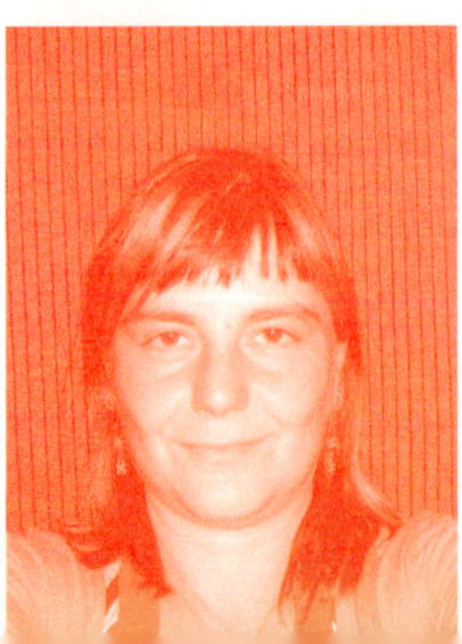

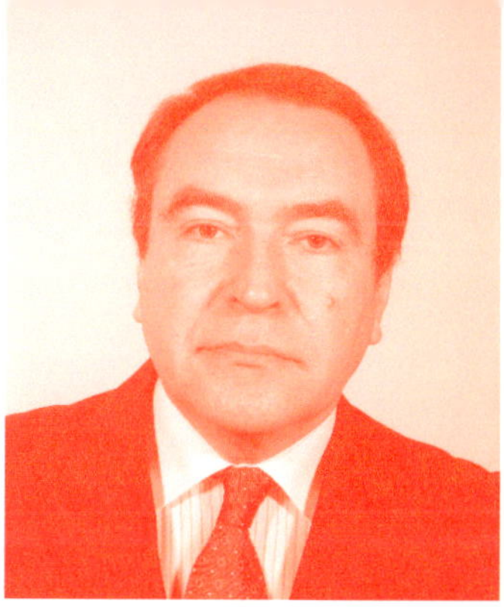
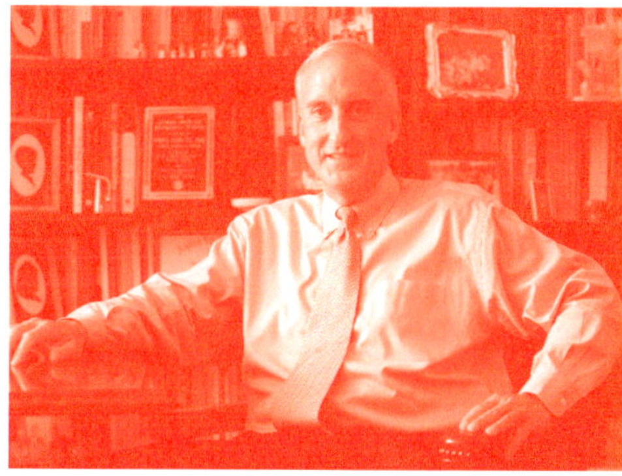
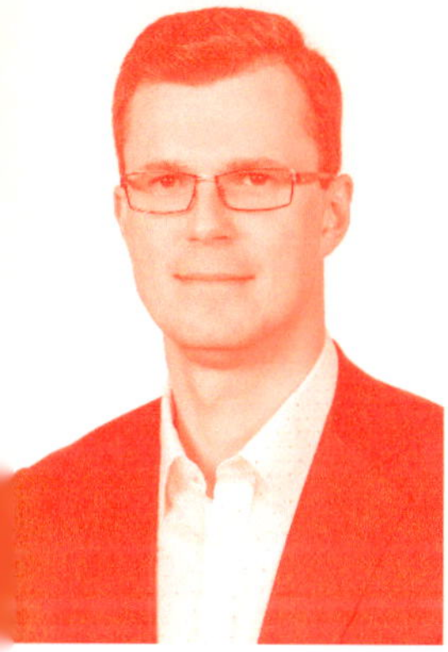
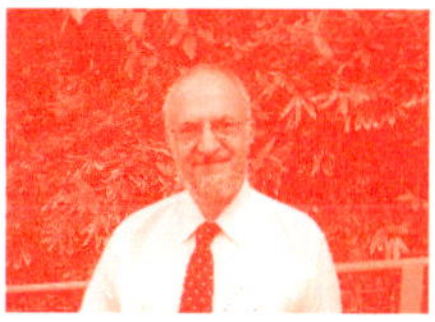
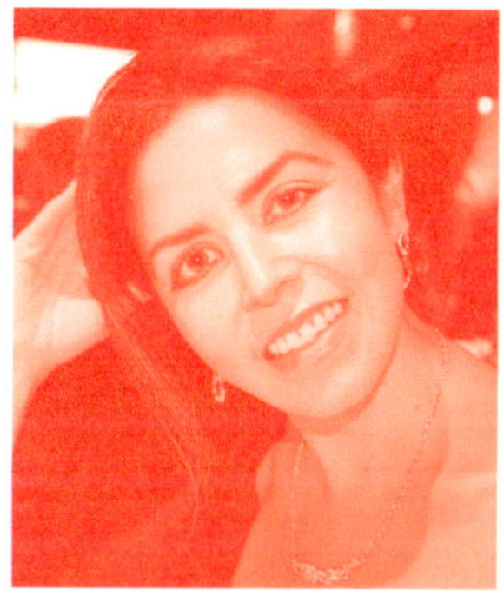

Supporting open minds since 2005

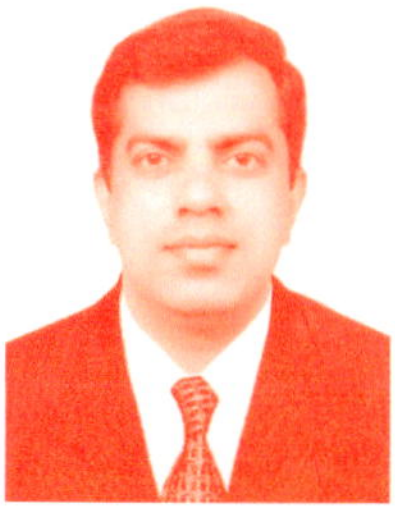
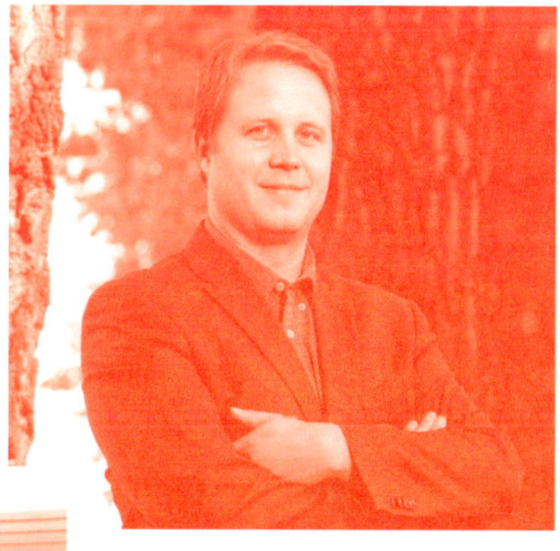
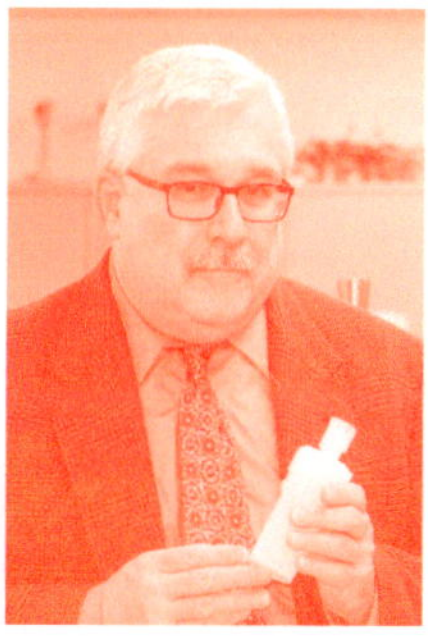
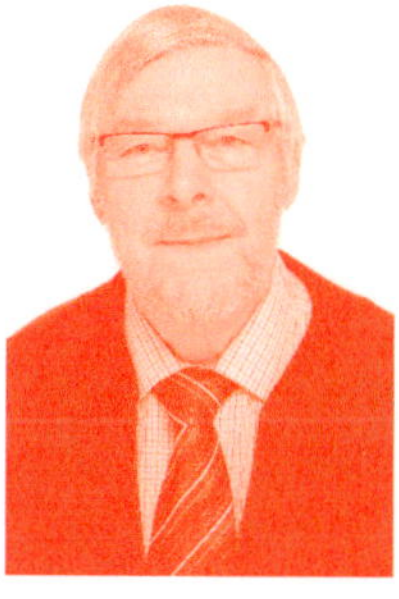
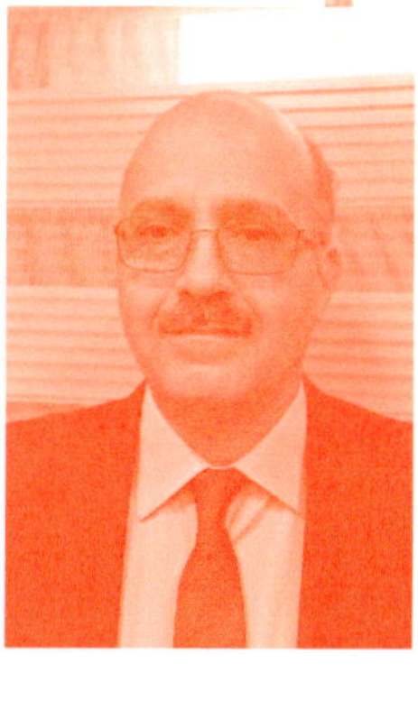
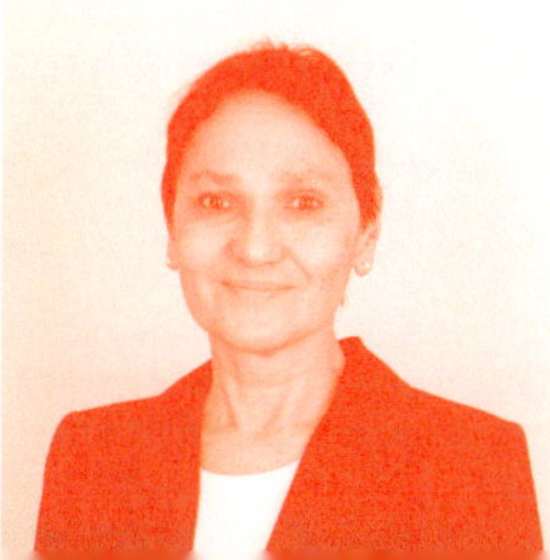
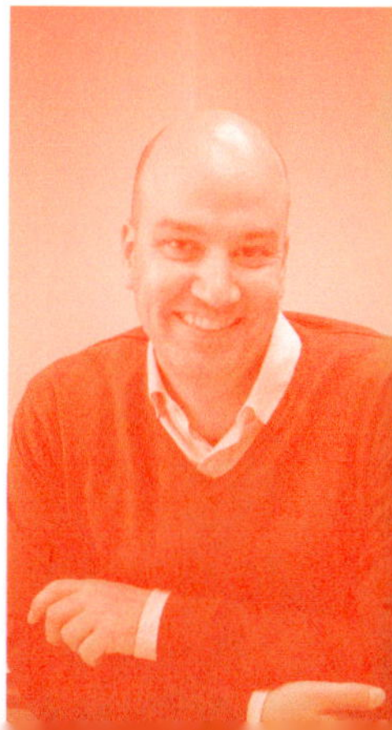

Dry Eye Syndrome - Modern Diagnostic Techniques and Advanced Treatments
http://dx.doi.org/10.5772/intechopen.94704
Edited by Felicia M. Ferreri

Contributors
José Luis Reyes Hernández, Alicia Vazquez-Mendoza, Danielle Vannan, Evelin G. Morales, Marisol I. González, Abraham Kayal, Sharita Siregar, Farideh Doroodgar, Sana Niazi, Shrinkhal, Rupal Verma, Anupam Singh, Mauricio Aguirre Baez, Rodrigo Castillo Iturria, Tri Wahyu

First published in London, United Kingdom, 2022 by IntechOpen
IntechOpen is the global imprint of INTECHOPEN LIMITED, registered in England and Wales, registration number: 11086078, 5 Princes Gate Court, London, SW7 2QJ, United Kingdom
Printed in Croatia

British Library Cataloguing-in-Publication Data
A catalogue record for this book is available from the British Library

Additional hard and PDF copies can be obtained from orders@intechopen.com

Dry Eye Syndrome - Modern Diagnostic Techniques and Advanced Treatments
Edited by Felicia M. Ferreri
p. cm.
Print ISBN 978-1-83969-454-7
Online ISBN 978-1-83969-455-4
eBook (PDF) ISBN 978-1-83969-456-1

For EU product safety concerns:
IN TECH d.o.o., Prolaz Marije Krucifikse Kozulić 3, 51000 Rijeka, Croatia, info@intechopen.com or visit our website at intechopen.com.

Meet the editor

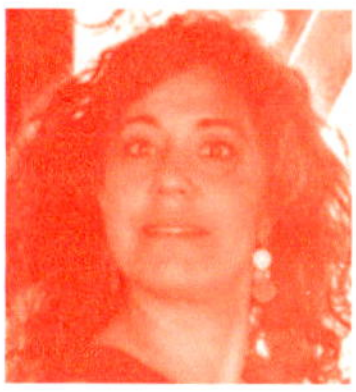

Felicia M. Ferreri graduated summa cum laude from the University of Messina, Italy, in 1998 and completed her ophthalmology residency at the Policlinico Universitario, Messina, in 2002. She interned at the Corneal Section of San Raffaele Hospital in Milan and at the Pediatric Ophthalmology Diseases Section of Hospital Careggi in Florence. She spent research periods at Virginio del Rocio hospital in Seville, San Carlos hospital in Madrid, the Royal Bolton Hospital in Manchester, and Universidade Fluminense in Rio de Janeiro. She served as co-investigator of many national and international clinical trials. Since 2002, she is an Assistant Professor in Ophthalmology at the University of Messina. Her research interests are in the areas of glaucoma, neuro-ophthalmology, pediatric ophthalmology, and cataract. She authored more than 50 scientific papers and edited two IntechOpen Books.

Contents

Preface

Dry eye syndrome, also known as keratoconjunctivitis sicca (KCS), is a disorder of the tear film caused by either tear deficiency or excessive tear evaporation.

In the latest decades, we gained a better and better understanding of dry eye syndrome. Early theories assumed that the syndrome was a mere consequence of aqueous tear insufficiency; today, it is classified as a multifactorial disorder caused by inflammation of the ocular surface and lacrimal glands, neurotrophic deficiency, and meibomian gland dysfunction.

The investigation on the composition and regulatory mechanisms of the preocular tear film was a milestone in scientific research about dry eye syndrome: the tear film, in fact, plays a key role in maintaining the corneal and conjunctival integrity, in protecting the eyes against infections, and, ultimately, in preserving visual acuity. Potential modification in the composition or structure of a tear film can have devastating effects, such as desiccation of the ocular surface and ulceration and perforation of the cornea; it is therefore not surprising that patients with dry eye syndrome are prone to potentially blinding infections, such as bacterial keratitis. Previous research works report an increased risk of complications in even common procedures (e.g., laser refractive surgery) in patients with dry eye syndrome.

Advances in dry eye syndrome research gave us a lot of hope in treating such a disease: today, in fact, we can get benefit from recent scientific discoveries to design more accurate diagnostic procedures as well as more advanced devices and effective medical treatments.

This book aims at illustrating the most recent research advances in the diagnosis as well as in the therapeutic strategies of dry eye. The book consists of seven chapters that cover a large spectrum of topics that can be of interest to professional ophthalmologists as well as students. Book chapters are from research groups located worldwide, thus highlighting the huge impact of dry eye syndrome on the field of ophthalmology and, perhaps, on many other medical disciplines to date. Each chapter has been carefully revised not only for scientific correctness but also for clarity: in this way, the proposed material is, in our opinion, accessible to a large, nonspecialist, audience, and thus, it can be regarded as a good entry point to the fascinating topic of dry eye syndrome.

The book is divided into two main sections

In the first section, the chapters describe the most recent diagnostic technique we can rely on today.

Chapter 1 entitled *Examination for Dry Eyes* extensively reviews dry eye diagnostic procedures. Ideally, all of the available tests could be performed at a single visit, but it is highly recommended the ophthalmologists follow a specific order in carrying out tests. Subjective symptoms often do not correlate with objective signs, and thus, laboratory tests, such as impression cytology, tear osmolarity, and ferning tests, greatly help in formulating a diagnosis. The most effective laboratory test, even if it might be too invasive for many patients, is the conjunctival biopsy, which analyzes specimens of epithelial layers and conjunctival stroma and is effective in identifying and counting the number of inflammatory cells.

Chapter 2 entitled *The Physiology of Tear Film* carefully points out the composition and functioning of the three-layer structure of the tear film, namely lipid, aqueous, and mucous layers. The chapter well clarifies that any disorder occurring in each of the three layers can affect the appearance of dry eye syndrome.

Chapter 3 is entitled *Lymphocytes in Dry Eye Disease* and highlights the role of the immune system in eye diseases, specifically in dry eye syndrome. In fact, modifications in immune cells, due to mechanical or chemical stimuli as well as infections, create, and magnify, immune responses that, in the long run, determine an injury of the ocular tissues.

Chapter 4 entitled *Diagnosis of Dry Eye* focuses on questionnaires, one of the most frequent techniques to diagnose dry eye syndrome. Questionnaires are relevant to measure parameters, such as the amount of tear secretion, tear clearance, tear volume, tear film stability, and tear evaporation, and quantify the degree of inflammation of the ocular surface and impact of inflammation on the daily lives of patients. Popular questionnaires are the Ocular Surface Disease Index (OSDI), Dry Eye Questionnaire (DEQ-5), Impact of Dry Eye on Everyday Living (IDEEL), and National Eye Institute's Visual Function Questionnaire (NEI VFQ-25).

The second section of the book is centered on the most recent, and promising, strategies to treat dry eye syndrome as well as on the potential, but often not fully elucidated, relationships among dry eye syndrome and other ocular diseases, such as glaucoma.

Chapter 5 entitled *Glaucoma and Dry Eye* discusses the side effects we might encounter in patients with glaucoma. Topical glaucoma treatments, in fact, cause chronic inflammations that severely affect the quantity and quality of tears: as a consequence, glaucoma medications may lead to the appearance of the syndrome or to its worsening. The chapter also surveys some recent treatments for patients with glaucoma proven to be effective in preserving the quality of the ocular surface.

Chapter 6 entitled *How Ocular Surface Disorder Affected Corneal Graft Survival* is about the role of dry eye syndrome in corneal graft failure. It is well-known, in fact, that inflammations, vascularization, and previous graft failure are high-risk factors in the rejection of cornea after a transplant. Corneas from patients with dry eye syndrome can activate an inflammatory process by increasing the number of T cells in the host, and this may predispose high rejection rates. Recently, HLA matching techniques have been applied in predicting graft survival rates in corneal transplants.

Finally, Chapter 7 entitled *Intense Pulse Laser Therapy and Dry Eye Disease* describes a recently approved therapy called IPL. IPL is a second-stage therapy that follows treatments based on ocular lubricants and relies on brief flashes of noncoherent light with a wavelength between 400 and 1200 nm.

Felicia M. Ferreri
BIOMORF Department,
University of Messina,
Messina, Italy

Section 1

Diagnosis of the Dry Eye Disease and Emerging Techniques

Chapter 1

Examination for Dry Eyes

Tri Wahyu

Abstract

Dry eye disease (DED) is a multifactorial disease of tears and ocular surface that results in various symptoms with the potential damage to the ocular surface. It can range from mild to severe signs and symptoms and may affect patient's quality of life. Various techniques and methods have been developed to evaluate DED for initial examination or regular follow up. The simple evaluations that can be performed in clinic include eyelid examination, tear break-up time, and ocular surface stainings; while the advanced ones may require certain devices or laboratory equipment. Careful and thorough examinations are important to guide the clinician to assess and evaluate dry eye.

Keywords: dry eye examination, ocular surface staining, tear film stability, tear volume, laboratory test

1. Introduction

Dry eye disease is one of the most commonly encountered problem in daily practice. It is the reason why a patient visits the eye care professional. Dry eye—as it was defined by the National Eye Institute (NEI)/Industry Workshop on Clinical Trials in Dry Eyes—is a disorder of the tear film due to tear deficiency or excessive evaporation, which causes damage to the interpalpebral ocular surface and is associated with symptoms of ocular discomfort [1]. In 2007, the International Dry Eye Workshop updated the original definition and classified dry eye as "multi-factorial disease of the tears and ocular surface that results in symptoms of discomfort, visual disturbance, and tear film instability with potential damage to the ocular surface. It is accompanied by increased osmolarity of the tear film and inflammation of the ocular surface" [2]. In 2017, the definition was revised, which centered on the clinical effects and associated signs as "multifactorial disease of the tears and ocular surface that results in symptoms of discomfort, visual disturbance, and tear film instability with potential damage to the ocular surface. It is accompanied by increased osmolarity of the tear film and inflammation of the ocular surface" [3].

Based on those definitions, dry eye symptoms can change from day to day and they may vary in every patient, from mild to severe ocular discomfort and visual disturbance. Dry eye disease can affect patients' quality of life. It is important for eye care professionals to recognize, diagnose, and treat DED; but, somehow DED can be puzzling since there is no consistent, well accepted, diagnostic test that is both readily available and reproducible [4]. When a patient comes in due to the symptoms that may suggest DED or for a routine examination, an eye care professional should do history taking comprehensively. Various diagnostic tests may be required to determine if the patient has DED due to aqueous deficient, evaporative, or both. In daily practice, tear-film and dry eye assessment are often performed in symptomatic patients. However, it must be kept in mind that dry eye symptoms and signs may be not well associated, as reported in previous studies [5–7].

2. History taking

A careful history taking is an important thing to perform in the first place to help the eye care professional in assessing dry eye correctly, including history of previous medication, long-term contact lens wear, ocular surface surgery, or systemic condition(s). Patients with dry eye often complain of eye discomfort or irritation, gritty or foreign body sensation, burning, tearing, stinging, intermittent sharp pain, redness, or/and photophobia. Visual disturbance may occur. Dry eye patients may have all, some, or none of these symptoms.

A clinician should also understand that dry eye symptoms increase with age, menopausal status, hormonal diseases, current smoking history, certain medications, and presence of pterygium are a few factors result in dry eye [4, 5, 8–10]. Noor et al. [7] found that there was a likelihood of shifting from preclinical dry eye towards DED and from normal towards predisposition to dry eye in older age.

There are many questionnaires available that can be used to utilize in assessing DED, such as National Eye Institute Visual Function Questionnaire-25 (NEV-VFQ-25) [11], Ocular Surface Disease Index (OSDI) [12], Standard Patient Evaluation of Dry Eye Questionnaire (DEQ-5) [13], and some others more. Every clinicians have their own preferences of questionniare.

3. Staining grading system

Visual acuity assessment (including best-corrected acuity), thorough eyelid and slit-lamp of anterior segment examinations are mandatory. Patients with dry eye often complain of blurred vision which improves with blinking or instillation of artificial tear.

Whilst taking patient's history, a clinician can examine the eyelids macroscopically. It can guide the clinician to evaluate if the patient has dry eye. Lagophthalmous, lid laxity, decreased frequency of blinking, and size of palpebral aperture. Malpositions of the eyelid have to be recognized (such as involutional or cicatrical ectropion, eversion of lacrimal punctum, dermatochalasis, full-thickness defects, inadequate lid closure due to previous eyelid surgical reconstruction) because these conditions can influence the tear turnover. Patient's history can guide the clinician to perform identify certain ocular manifestations under careful and focused slit-lamp examination.

3.1 Slit-lamp biomicroscopy

Under the slit-lamp biomicroscopy, a clinician should evaluate anatomical structures of the lid, including the alterations of lid margins and eyelashes. The alterations of the lid margins include hyperaemia, telangiectasia, thickening, scarring, keratinization, ulceration, tear debris, abnormalities of the meibomian orifices, metaplasia, character of expressed meibomian secretions; while for the eyelashes, the alterations include misdirection (trichiasis), malposition (dystichiasis), encrustations, collarettes [14–16]. Careful evaluation of meibomian gland is important since its dysfunction is the most frequent cause of evaportive DED and is often symtomatic [17–19]. Evaluate if the meibomian gland orifices are plugged or obstructed and/or change in its secretion.

Tear film should be evaluated for mucus, debris, or meibomian foam. Decreased tear meniscus is often a sign of dry eye. Normally, a patient with normal tear production has tear meniscus height of 0.2–0.5 mm; but in patient with dry eye, it is usually less than 0.25 mm or absent [4, 14, 15, 20, 21].

Ocular manifestations in mild to moderate dry eye may conjunctival hyperaermia, with or without corneal epithelial erosions; or these signs may not present in some mild cases. In severe forms of the disease, conjunctival scarring or conjunctivochalasis and/or corneal complications may occur. Filamentary keratitis, persistent epithelial defects, ulceration, and even corneal perforation can complicate the course [14, 15, 22]. Corneal staining may be required to evaluate the severity of its defects.

There are several tests that can be performed to confirm the diagnosis of dry eye and to evaluate the severity of the disease. The tests can measure the following parameters: (1) stability of the tear film as related to its break-up time (TBUT); (2) tear production (Schirmer, fluorescein clearance, and tear osmolarity); and (3) ocular surface disease (corneal stains and impression cytology). There is no clinical test to confirm the diagnosis of evaporative dry eye [21, 23].

3.2 Staining of the ocular surface

Epithelial damage to the exposed ocular surface can be evaluated with vital stainings. Staining of the cornea occurs commonly in inferior part, often more in nasal and temporal areas. Corneal epithelial defect, erosions, filaments, or punctuates can be seen in dry eye. Staining of the bulbar conjunctiva occurs over a wedge-shaped zone nasally and temporally, and in advanced dry eye may become confluent; but in milder forms of dry eye, it may be present in the absence of corneal stain [23].

3.2.1 Fluorscein

Fluorscein staining is a basic and standard method to evaluate ocular surface damage. Commonly, every clinician is able to perform this examination in daily practice. The orange-dyed fluorescein strip is wetted with a sterile drop of saline and then is applied to tarsal or bulbar conjunctiva. Excess fluid is shaken from the strip prior to application. The dye will distribute over ocular surface after blinking. Under slit-lamp examination using cobalt-blue filter, the orange dye will turn into fluoresces green in the damaged area. Common characteristic distribution of this test is confined to the exposed intrapalpebral area of the ocular surface, but the staining may extend to unexposed area in severe case.

In the case of perforation, aqueous from the anterior chamber will leak out of the eye and mix with the tear film. The fluorescein dye around the perforated area will be diluted by this leak and the leak will appear bright green (Seidel test).

3.2.2 Rose bengal

Rose bengal is a synthetic fluorescein derivative, also perhaps referred to as bengal rose and also known as a Chemical Index (C.I.) Acid Red 94 [24]. It has the ability to bind to epithelial cells that are uncoated by certain proteins (mainly mucin) and presents high cell toxicity [25]. The instillation of this dye causes stinging or pain, particularly in DED patients, and it may be disliked by some patients; thus topical anesthesia is best instilled first to limit stinging sensation. Although rose bengal had been thought to be a vital dye, staining dead or degenerating cells, it is known that rose bengal normally stains healthy cells [26, 27].

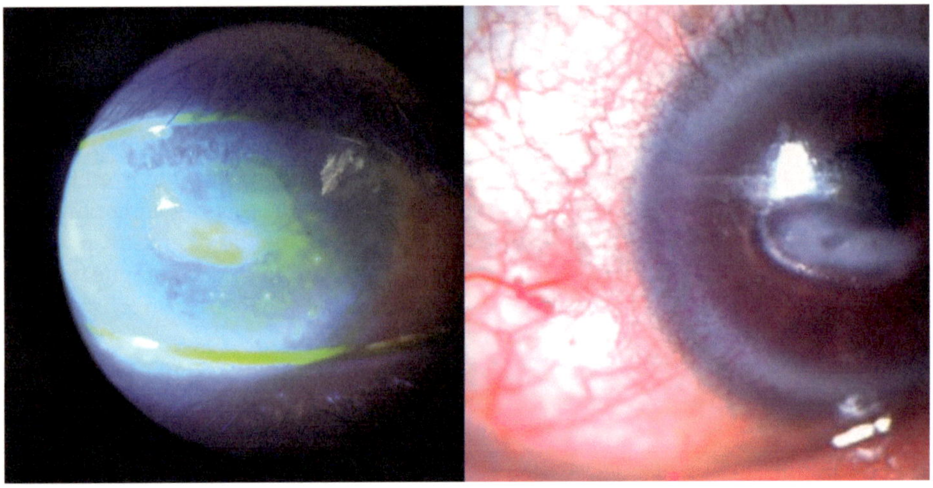

Figure 1.
Left: Fluorescein staining shows large defect in central cornea with discrete punctate staining all over cornea; right: Rose bengal staining in the same patient.

Under slit-lamp with a white light, rose bengal staining can revealed discrete or confluent punctuate in damaged area of cornea and visible bulbar conjunctiva which can be seen as red dots (**Figure 1**). But there are disadvantages in using rose bengal in addition to pain on instillation. Although bulbar conjunctival staining is demonstrated well against the white background provided by the sclera, the dye is difficult to see on the cornea against the background of a dark iris [23]. Another disadvantage of rose bengal is its toxicity, including decreasing the chance to recover herpes viruses in human cell cultures [25].

3.2.3 Lissamine green

Lissamine green is a synthetically produced organic acid dye with two aminophenyl group and it has been used as a substitute for rose bengal since it has similar laboratory and clinical staining properties, also it is a less toxic stain and less stinging upon instillation [25, 28].

	Fluorescein	**Rose Bengal**	**Lissamine Green**
Discomfort (pain/stinging)	No	Yes	No
Staining normal/healthy cells	No	Yes	No
Staining dead or degenerated cells	No	Yes	Yes
Clinical means	Disruption of cellular junctions and increased membrane permeability	Loss of insufficient protection by ocular surface mucin	Cell degeneration and death (unprotected by ocular mucin or glyco-calyx)
Slit-lamp filter	Cobalt-blue	White light or green barrier filter	Red barrier filter

Adapted from [29].

Table 1.
Comparison of ocular surface stainings.

Lissamine green is a vital dye that stains ocular surface epithelial cells that are unprotected by mucin or glycocalyx, as well as cells that have been damaged, and it does not stain healthy cells or damage them [28–30]. In patient with red eyes, lissamine green could provide better staining visualization than rose bengal.

The use of ocular staining mentioned above is helpful in assessing the integrity of the ocular surface epithelium. These tests are easy to perform in daily clinical practice in-office setting. The clinician can choose one of these staining to assess dry eye based on the availability of the equipment in the clinic. Fluorescein impregnated strips are preferred due to their availability and simplicity of use; while rose bengal and/or lissamine may not always be available in some eye care facilities. **Table 1** helps the clinician to compare these three stainings. Significant staining of the conjunctiva with rose bengal or lissamine green is most common in severe dry eye to Sjögren's syndrome [29].

4. Staining grading systems

Staining grading systems remain an essential element of ocular examination and allow the clinician to record the level of ocular surface staining and evaluate the severity of dry eye. The three most common grading systems are: (1) the van Bijsterveld grading system (uses rose bengal staining of the conjunctiva and cornea); (2) the Oxford grading scheme (uses fluorescein, rose bengal, or lissamine green of the conjunctiva and cornea); and (3) and the NEI Workshop system (uses fluorescein staining to grade the cornea and rose bengal to grade the conjunctiva) [29].

The van Bijstervel grading system is the first proposed system to grade three areas in each eye: the nasal and temporal bulbar conjunctiva and the cornea (**Figure 2**). The intensity of the staining is graded on scale 0 (no staining), 1 (sparsely scattered staining), 2 (densely scattered), and 3 (confluent staining). The maximum score for each eye is 9. Staining score of 3 or higher is considered abnormal.

The Oxford grading scheme uses a chart consisting of a series of panels labeled A to E in order of increasing severity of staining (**Figure 3**). Staining is represented by punctate dots and increases by 1 log unit between panel A and B and by ½ log unit between each subsequent panel (B to E).

The NEI Workshop grading system divides cornea into five areas and conjunctiva into six areas for each eye (**Figure 4**). The scale of 0 to 3 is used for the grading, according to the intensity of fluorescein staining. The maximum staining score for the cornea is 15, and for conjunctiva, the maximum score is 18. The values above 3 is considered abnormal for cornea or conjunctiva in each eye.

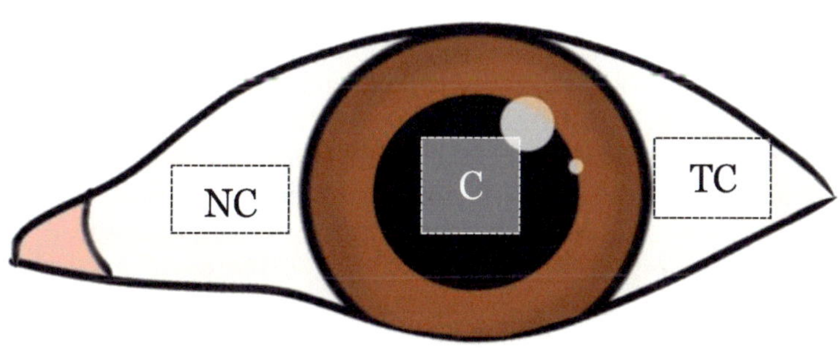

Figure 2.
The van Bijsterveld grading system. The exposed nasal and temporal conjunctiva (NC and NT, respectively) and cornea (C) are graded on scale: 0 (no staining) to 3 (confluent staining), with maximum score is 9.

A	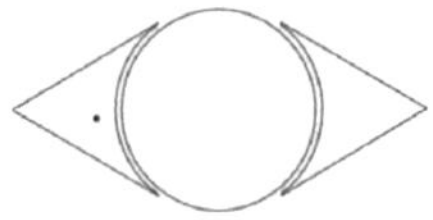	Equal to or less than picture A	Log: 0	Grade 0 (absent)
B	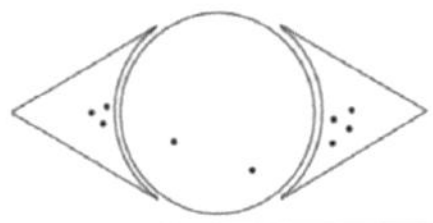	Equal to or less than picture B, greater than A	Log: 1	Grade 1 (minimal)
C	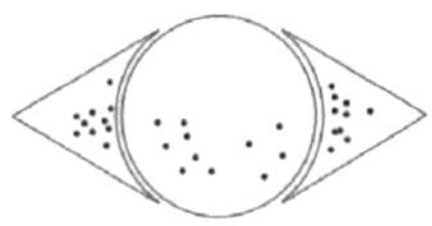	Equal to or less than picture C, greater than B	Log: 1.5	Grade 2 (mild)
D	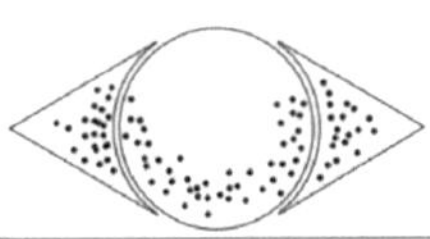	Equal to or less than picture D, greater than C	Log: 2.0	Grade 3 (moderate)
E	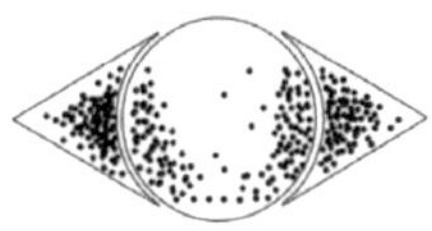	Equal to or less than picture E, greater than D	Log: 2.5	Grade 4 (marked)
>E		Greater than picture E	Log: >2.5	Grade 5 (severe)

Figure 3.
The Oxford grading scheme. Staining is represented by punctate dots. (adapted from Bron AJ, Evan VE, smith JA. Grading of corneal and conjunctival staining in the context of other dry eye tests. Cornea 2003;22(7):640–650).

4.1 Laboratory tests

Lack of stability in the tear film can be seen in aqueous deficient, evaporative, or both type of dry eye. It may also occur in the setting of a poor blink rate or epithelial irregularity [30]. There are several numbers of tools designed to evaluate tear film stability to help clinician or researcher to assess and support the diagnosis of DED.

4.1.1 Tear break-up time (TBUT)

Tear break-up time was first introduced by Norn in 1969 and remains the most frequently used diagnostic test to evaluate tear film stability [31]. It measures the time between a complete blink and the first appearance of a dry spot on the ocular surface using fluorscein. Right after applying the fluorescein strip on to the ocular surface, and under cobalt blue filter in slit-lamp biomicroscopy, patient is asked to blink completely and hold the eye open (avoid blinking). The clinician should observe the first dry spots appear on his/her ocular surface. Normally, dry spot(s) will appear after 10 seconds.

The TBUT less than 10 seconds is considered as a cut-off score for the diagnosis of dry eye, with values of 5–10 seconds are considered marginal and less than 5 seconds indicate the dry eye symptoms [31–34]. But, the threshold for Asian patients may be set much lower as many Asians with TBUT between about 7–10 seconds do not have dry eye symptoms [35]. Some studies suggest that healthy Asian subjects

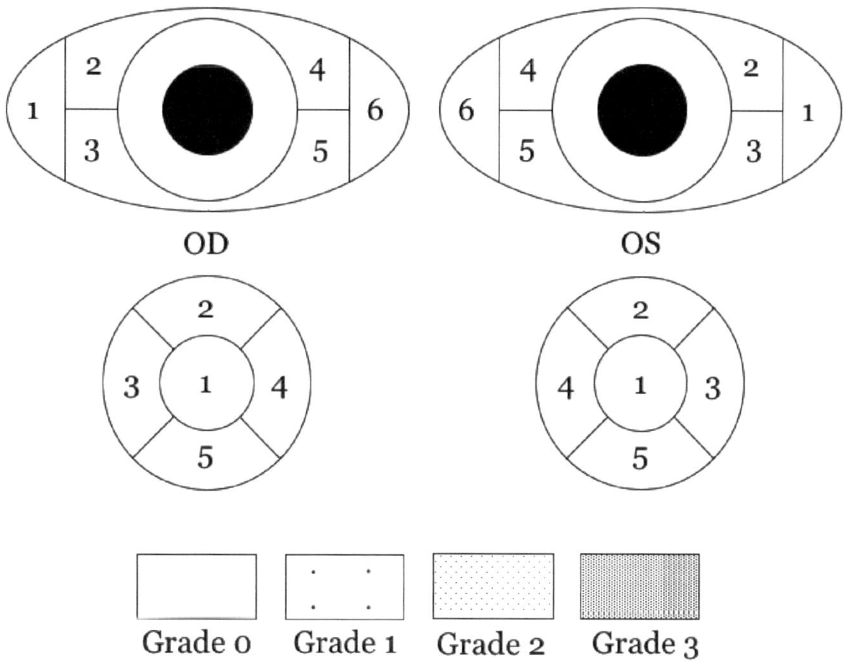

Figure 4.
The NEI scale system for grading fluorescein staining which divides the corneal and conjunctival surfaces. The conjunctival surface is divided into 6 areas and the corneal surface is divided into 5 areas. A standardized grading system of 0 to 3 is used for each of areas on cornea and conjunctiva.

have an 11–24% shorter TBUT than non-Asians [35, 36]. It hypothesized that the tear lipid layer is not able to efficiently perform its usual expansion and compression during a blink in an eye with a small palpebral aperture size (Asian), resulting in a less stable tear film [37].

4.1.2 Non-invasive break-up time (NIBUT)

This technique was first introduced by Mengher et al. in 1983 and is defined as 'the time taken in seconds between the last complete blink and the appearance of the first random disturbance of a grid' [38, 39]. The NIBUT test can be performed using several device options, such as topography, keratography, or Placido disc video-keratography. Tear break-up time is considered when the reflected mires become distorted.

Mengher et al. [38] reported a NIBUT value of 47.9 seconds (range of four to 214 seconds), but Mohidin et al [36] reported lower NIBUT value (15.8 ± 9.4 seconds, range of 4.2 to 48.6 seconds). Sharanjeet-Kaur et al. [40] reported that NIBUT values for normal Malays and Chinese were 7.74 ± 3.34 seconds and 7.15 ± 3.38 seconds respectively. Generally, in normal population, NIBUT is longer than TBUT, with range of four to 214 seconds (median 4–19 seconds); and in patients with DED, NIBUT and TBUT values are almost the same (the cut-off values for positive finding can be as low as 2.7 seconds for automated algorithms and up to 10 seconds for subjective observation techniques) [41].

4.2 Tear volume

The aim of tear volume assessment is to measure the quantity of tear film produced by lacrimal gland and conjunctiva.

4.2.1 Schirmer's test

The Schirmer's test is the most common examination performed whenever there is a suspicion of inadequate tear secretion. The test was named after Schirmer who brought the test forward for the first time in 1903 [42]. Basically, without anesthesia, the test measures total (basic and reflex) tear secretion, as with anesthesia it measures basic tear secretion devoid of reflex component [43, 44]. This test remains as the most common test used for tear quantity assessment [45]. It can be divided into Schirmer I and Schirmer II test.

The Schirmer I test is performed using strip that is folded from one end and inserted into the lower conjunctival sac at the junction of lateral and middle thirds, avoiding touching the cornea. After five minutes, the length of wetted strip is recorded. Fifteen minutes later, after instillation of topical anesthesia, the strip is placed again over the same point in the same patient for five minutes. The Schirmer II test measure reflex secretion of lacrimal gland. The procedure of this test is as the same as Schirmer I test with topical anesthesia and nasal mucosa is irritated with a cotton-tiped applicator prior to measuring tear production. The result is recorded after 5 minutes. Normally, the length of wetted strip is around 10 mm or greater and if the length is less than 5 mm, it indicates symptomatic tear deficient; but Schirmer's test values less or equal to 10 mm have greater diagnostic value and indicate hyposecretion [22, 46–50].

4.2.2 Phenol red thread test

The phenol red thread (PRT) test was invented by Hamano in 1982 and developed to overcome the disadvantage of Schirmer's test including variable results, poor repeatibility, and low sensitivity in detecting dry eyes [44, 51–53]. The test uses a special cotton thread impregnated with phenol red (a pH-sensitive indicator). The procedure is performed in the similar manners to Schirmer test, which the thread is folded at the end and inserted into the lower conjunctival sac and it will absorb the tears that contact with it. The color of this thread will change from yellow to red over the pH range of normal tears. The result is recorded after 15 seconds, much shorter than Schirmer's test. The PRT is almost comparable with Schirmer's test and it has advantages including simpler and more comfortable to the patient and can also be performed in children [54].

4.3 Laboratory tests

Conjunctival biopsy may be one of the best methods to investigate and evaluate the ocular surface condition, which offers specimens of epithelial layers and conjunctival stroma to be examined under light or electron microscopy, cytology, and immunohistochemical analyses. These techniques may allow identification and counting of inflammatory cells and analysis of cell membrane markers, intracyto-plasmic cells, or extracellular matrix components [55]. But, of all methods mentioned above, conjunctival biopsy is an invasive technique that may cause discomfort to the patient.

4.3.1 Impression cytology

Impression cytology (IC) refers to the application of cellulose acetate filter to the ocular surface to remove the superficial layers of the ocular surface epithelium [56]. The analysis techniques used in this method vary, depend on the purpose and the equipment availability in eye care facility. The simplest analysis technique remains light microscopy, in which epithelial and goblet cells can be well visualized through hemtoxylin and periodic acid Schiff (PAS) staining. Other techniques include electron microscopy, immunohistochemistry, flow cytometry, and RT-PCR/PCR.

The RT-PCR was used in IC specimens as early as 1994 and identified inflammatory cytokins in conjunctival specimens from Sjögren's syndrome eyes [57].

4.3.2 Tear osmolarity

Tear osmolarity is the most accurate method to diagnose DED. Tear hyperosmolarity is considered as pathogenic factor causing ocular surface inflammation, symptoms, and tissue damage which can lead to DED. This condition can occur in many situations including insufficient tear production, meibomian gland dysfunction, and exposure. There is a commercially available objective point of care test (TearLab Osmolarity System; TearLab, San Diego, California) that can measure the osmolarity of a 50-nL tear sample and is easier to use [30, 58, 59]. A reading of 308 mOsms/L or greater indicates tear osmolarity disruption. This test must be completed quickly to avoid any evaporation of tear sample. Although reproducible, this test is difficult to perform in clinic setting.

4.3.3 Ferning test

Tear ferning test is a simple test for tear film quality. This test requires capillary tubes, spatula, or glass rods to collect tear from the lower tear meniscus (about 5–20 μl). The collected tear is applied to a glass slide and evaluated under light or digital microscope with various magnifications (40-100x). In DED, the delicate fronded pattern becomes fragmented or broken up and irregular and the appearances can be graded into type I and II (healthy tear film) and type III and IV (increasing degrees of dry eye) [14, 60].

5. Assessing the dry eye

The diagnosis of dry eye depends on the results of several of tests mentioned above, which ideally could be performed at a single clinic visit. It is important to keep in mind that a clinician should carry out the test in an appropriate order. **Table 2** suggests a suitable order for diagnostic test, although there are various and informal data to justify a particular sequence of the tests. Some of the standard tests are specific for subgroup of the disease (**Table 3**). **Table 4** helps the clinician to grade the severity of the DED.

1. Patient history (a symptom-oriented questionnaire may be needed).
2. Measure UCVA and BCVA.
3. Observe eyelid and its skin appearance, including upper and lower lid positions.
4. Measure blink rate.
5. Tear-film break-up time with fluorescein
6. Ocular surface staining
7. Schirmer test with/without anesthesia
8. Slit lamp xamination of the eyelid margins, meibomian gland orifices with expression of meibomian secretion, and anterior segments.

Table 2.
Practical sequence of dry eye tests.

- Schirmer test evaluates the aqueous phase secretion.
- Altered meibomian gland status can be characteristic of evaporative dry eye. Other conditions that can be the signs of evaporative dry eye include:
    - changes in tear composition (lack of lipid content; primary type: lack of gland and distichiasis; secondary type: bleharitis and MGD);
    - abnormalities of eyelids, reduced blinking rate or incomplete blinking (office workers, Parkinsonism, and schizophrenia);
    - ocular surface irregularities;
    - contact lens wear.
- Tear-film hyperosmolarity is considered a key pathological factor, both in aqueous tear-deficient and in evaporative dry eye disease.

Adapted from Módis and Szalai [22].

Table 3.
Practical applications of several test for assessing DED.

	Dry Eye Severity Level			
	1	2	3	4
Discomfort, severity, and frequency	Mild and/or episodic; occurs under enviromental stress	Moderate episodic or chronic, strees or no stress	Severe frequent or constant without stress	Severe and/or disabling and constant
Visual symptoms	None or episodic mild fatigue	Annoying and/or activity-limiting episodic	Annoying, chronic and/ or constant, limiting activity	Constant and/or possibly dissabling
Conjunctival injection	None to mild	None to mild	Mild or not present	Mild to moderate
Corneal staining (severity/location)	None to mild	Variable	Marked central	N/A
Cornea/tear signs	None to mild	Mild debris, decreased meniscus	Filamentary keratitis, mucus clumping, increased tear debris	Filamentary keratitis, mucus clumping, increased tear debris, ulceration
Lid/meibomian glands	MGD variably present	MGD variably present	MGD frequent	Trichiasis, keratinization, symblepharon
TBUT (seconds)	Variable	≤ 10	≤ 5	Immediate
Schirmer score (mm/5 minutes)	Variable	≤ 10	≤ 5	≤ 2

Table 4.
The severity grading scheme for dry eye disease.

Despite the wide use in clinical practice, standard tests for assessing DED and ocular surface disorders (including history taking and symptoms recording, TBUT, meibomian gland testing, ocular surface saining, and Schirmer's testing) have shown poor repeatability and lack of efficacy [22, 57]. Moreover, it is well know that subjective symptoms often do not correlate with objective signs. Additional exploratory technique may be required to assess DED and evaluate the severity of the disease. The laboratory test may be required in patient who have subjective complaint

• Subjective description of oral symptoms
• Subjective description of ocular symptoms
• Objective signs of oral dryness, determined by unstimulated salivary flow rate and/or Saxon test
• Objective signs of ocular dryness, diagnosed on the basis of a reduced Schirmer test result, reduced TBUT, and/or positive ocular surface staining
• Histopathological evidence of infiltrating lymphocytes in minor salivary glands
• Evidence of serum autoantibodies, especially antibodies to Ro(SSA) or La(SSB) antigens

Table 5.
Diagnosis criteria for Sjögren's syndrome.

that is not identified as dry eye (such as fluctuating vision) but do not show a lot of ocular finding such as corneal staining or any other marked conditions.

Patient with xerostomia in addition to dry eye must be investigated for the possible presence of Sjögren's syndrome. The revised criteria of the European-American Consensus Group for the diagnosis of Sjögren's syndrome are summarized in **Table 5**. The diagnosis of Sjögren's syndrome is made if four of the six criteria are fulfilled. If SSA/SSB diagnostic testing is negative, a positive ANA (antinuclear antibody) test or positive rheumatoid factors may be indicative [15].

6. Conclusion

Careful and thorough examinations help the clinician to assess and evaluate dry eye disease. Various examinations are available, but the clinicians must adjust the examination to the available tools or equipments in their facilities. Ocular surface staining is the simplest test that can be performed in every clinic. If the case is complicated with or without underlying disease and needs further examniations, a clinician should refer to higher facility or dry eye specialist.

Acknowledgements

Author would like to acknowledge Susi Heryati, Angga Fajriansyah, Arief Mustaram, Patriotika Muslima, and Elfa Ali Idrus as supervisors in Infection and Immunology Division, Department of Ophthalmology, Cicendo National Eye Hospital, Bandung, Indonesia.

Conflict of interest

The author declares that there is no conflict of interest in this work.

Appendices and nomenclature

ANA	antinuclear antibody
BCVA	best-corrected visual acuity
C.I.	chemical index
DED	dry eye disease
DEQ-5	Standard Patient Evaluation for Dry Eye Questionnaire
IC	impression cytology

MGD	meibomian gland dysfunction
mOsm	milliosmole
NEI	National Eye Institute
NEV-VFQ-25	National Eye Institute Function Questionnaire-25
NIBUT	non-invasive break-up time
OSDI	Ocular Surface Disease Index
PAS	periodic acid Schiff
PCR	polymerase chain reaction
pH	power of hydrogen
PRT	phenol red thread
RT-PCR	reverse transcription polymerase chain reaction
SSA	anti-Sjögren's syndrome type A
SSB	anti-Sjögren's syndrome type B
TBUT	tear break-up time
UCVA	uncorrected visual acuity

Author details

Tri Wahyu
Sawangan Eye Clinic Depok, West Java, Indonesia

*Address all correspondence to: tri.why89@gmail.com

References

[1] Lemp MA. Report of the National eye Institute/industry workshop on clinical trials in dry eyes. CLAO J. 1995;21: 221-232

[2] [No author listed]. The definition and classification of dry eye disease: Report of the definition and classification subcommittee of the international dry eye workshop. Ocul Surf. 2007;5(2):75-92

[3] Craig JP, Nichols KK, Akpek EK, Caffery B, Dua HS, Joo CK, et al. TFOS DEWS II definition and classification report. Ocul Surf. 2017;15:276-283. DOI: 10.1016/j.jtos.2017.05.008

[4] Zeev MSB, Miller DD, Latkany R. Diagnosis of dry eye disease and emerging technologies. Clin Ophthalmol. 2014;8:581-590 DOI: 10.2147/OPTH.S45444

[5] Schein OD, Tielsch JM, Munõz B, Bandeen-Roche K, West S. Relation between signs and symptoms of dry eye in the elderly. Ophthalmology 1997;104:1395-1401

[6] McCarty CA, Bansal AK, Livingston PM, Stanislavsky YL, Taylor HR. The epidemiology of dry eye in Melbourne, Australia. Ophthalmology 1998;105:1114-1119

[7] Noor NA, Rahayu T, Gondhowiardjo TD. Prevalence of dry eye and its subtypes in an elderlu population with cataracts in Indonesia. Clin Ophthalmol. 2020; 14:2143-2150. DOI: 10.1097/00003226-200208000-00009

[8] de Paiva CS. Effects of aging in dry eye. Int Ophthlamol Clin. 2017 Spring;57(2): 47-64. DOI: 10.1097/IIO.0000000000000170

[9] Sharma A, Hindman HB. Aging: A predisposition to dry eyes. J Ophthalmol. 2014;2014:781683. DOI: 10.1155/2014/781683

[10] Lee AJ, Lee J, Saw SM, Gazzard G, Koh D, Widjadja D, et al. Prevalence and risk factors associated with dry eye symptoms: A population based study in Indonesia. Br J Ophthalmol. 2002;86:1347-1351

[11] Nichols KK, Mitchell GL, Zadnik K. Performance and repeatability of the NEI-VFQ-25. Cornea 2002;21(6):578-583. DOI: 10.10970/01.ICO.0000016353.01275.23

[12] Schiffman RM, Christianson MD, Jacobsen G, Hirsch JD, Reis BL. Reliability and validity of the ocular surface disease index. Arch Ophthalmol. 2000;18:615-621. DOI: 10.1001/archopht.118.615

[13] Chalmers RL, Begley CG, Caffery B. Validation of the 5-item dry eye questionnaire (DEQ-5): Discrimination across self-assessed severity and aqueous tear deficient dry eye diagnoses. Contact Lens and Anterior Eye 2010;33:55-60. DOI: 10.1016/j.clae.2009.12.010

[14] Kaercher T, Anthony JB. Classification and diagnosis of dry eye. Dev Ophthalmol. 2008;41:36-53.

[15] Messmer EM. The pathophysiology, diagnosis, and treatment of dry eye disease. Dtsch Arztebl Int. 2015;112:71-82. DOI: 10.3238/arztebl.2015.0071

[16] Chhadva P, Goldhardt R, Galor A. Meibomian gland disease: The role of gland dysfunction in dry eye disease. Ophthalmology 2017;124(11):S20-S26. DOI: 10.1016/j.ophtha.2017.05.031

[17] Yokoi N, Mossa F, Tiffany JM, Bron AJ. Assessment of meibomian gland function in dry eye using meibometry. Arch Ophthalmol.

1999;117:723-729. DOI: 10.1001/archopht.117.6.723

[18] Boudouin C, Messmer EM, Aragona P, Geerling G, Akova YA, Benítez-del-Castillo J, et al. Revisiting the vicious circle of dry eye disease: A focus on the pathophysiology of meibomian gland dysfunction. Br J Ophthalmol. 2016;100: 300-306. DOI: 10.1136/ojophthalmol-2015-307415

[19] Dell SJ, Gaster RN, Barbarino SC, Cunningham DN. Prospective evaluation of intense pulsed light and meibomian gland expression efficacy on relieving signs and symptoms of dry eye disease due to meibomian gland dysfunction. Clin Ophthalmol. 2017;11:817-827. DOI: 10.2147/OPTH.S130706

[20] Mainstone JC, Bruce AS, Golding TR. Tear meniscus measurement in the diagnosis of dry eye. Curr Eye Res. 1996;15:653-661. DOI: 10.3109/02713689609008906

[21] Salmon JF. Kanski's Clinical Ophthalmology. 9th ed. Edinburgh: Elsevier; 2020. p. 156-165. DOI: 9780702077135

[22] Módis L, Szalai E. Dry eye diagnosis and management. Expert Rev Ophthalmol. 2011;6(1):67-79. DOI: 10.1586/eop.10.89

[23] Bron AJ. Diagnosis of dry eye. Surv Ophthalmol. 2001;45(Suppl 2):S221-S226. DOI: 10.1016/s0039-6257(00)00201-0

[24] Doughty MJ. Rose bengal staining as an assessment of ocular surface damage and recovery in dry eye disease—a review. Contact Lens and Anterior Eye 2013; 36:272-280. DOI: 10.106/j.clae.2013.07.008

[25] Machado LM, Castro RS, Fontes BM. Staining patterns in dry eye syndrome: Rose bengal versus lissamine green. Cornea 2009;28:732-734. DOI: 10.1097/ICO.0b013e3181930c03

[26] Feenstra RP, Tseng SC. Comparison of fluorescein and rose bengal staining. Ophthalmology 1992;99(4):605-617. DOI: 10.106/s0161-6420(92)31947-5

[27] Feenstra RPG, Tseng SCG. What is actually stained by rose bengal?. Arch Ophthalmol 1992;110(7):984-993. DOI: 10.1001/archopht.1992.01080190090035

[28] Hamrah P, Alipour F, Jiang S, Sohn JH, Foulks GN. Optimizing evaluation of lissamine green parameters for ocular surface staining. Eye 2011;25:1429-1434. DOI: 10.1038/eye.2011.184

[29] Nelson JD. In-office diagnostic tests for dry eye disease. In: Asbell PA, Lemp MA, editors. Dry Eye Disease: The Clinician's Guide to Diagnosis and Treatment. New York: Thieme; 2006. p. 34-46. DOI: 10.1055/b-002-51025

[30] Kloosterboer A, Dermer HI, Galor A. Diagnostic tests in dry eye. Expert Rev Ophthalmol. 2019;14(4-5):237-246. DOI: 10.1080/17469899.2019.1657833

[31] Sweeney DF, Millar TJ, Raju SR. Tear film stability. Experimental Eye Research 2013;117:28-38. DOI: 10.106/j.exer.2013.08.010

[32] Wang MTM, Murphy PJ, Blades KJ, Craing JP. Comparison of non-invasive tear film stability measurement techniques. Clin Exp Optom. 2018;101:13-17. DOI: 10.1111/cxo.12546

[33] Plugfelder SC, Tseng SCG, Sanabria O, Kell H, Garcia CG, Felix C, et al. Evaluation of subjective assessments and objective diagnostic tests for diagnosing tear-film disorders known to cause ocular irritation. Cornea 1998;17(1):38-56. DOI: 10.1097/00003226-199801000-00007

[34] O'Brien PD, Collum LMT. Dry eye: Diagnosis and current treatment strategies. Current Allergy and Asthma Reports 2004;4:314-319. DOI: 10.1007/s11882-004-0077-2

[35] Mohidin N, Bay TC, Yap M. Non-invasive tear break-up time in normal Malays. Clin Exp Optom. 2002;85(1):37-41. DOI: 10.1111/j.1444-0938.2002.tb03070.x

[36] Yeh TN, Graham AD, Lin MC. Relationships among tear film stability, osmolarity, and dryness symptoms. Optom Vis Sci. 2015;92(9):e264-e272. DOI: 10.1097/OPX.0000000000000649

[37] Wang H, Seger KR, Yang S, Xing X. The role of ethnicity versus environment in tear film stability: a pilot study. Contact Lens and Anterior Eye 2019;42:553-556. DOI: 10.106/j.clae.2019.04.015

[38] Mengher LS, Bron AJ, Tonge SR, Gilbert DJ. A non-invasive instrument for clinical assessment of the pre-corneal tear film stability. Curr Eye Res. 1985; 4(1):1-7. DOI: 10.3109/02713688508999960

[39] Mengher LS, Pandher KS, Bron AJ. Non-invasive tear film break-up time: sensitivity and specificty. Acta Ophthalmol. 1986;64:441-444. DOI: 10.111/j.1755-3768.1986.tb06950.x

[40] Sharanjeet-Kaur, Ho CY, Mutalib HA, Ghazali AR. The relationship between tear ferning patterns and non-invasive tear break-up time in normal Asian population. Journal of Optometry 2016;9:175-181. DOI: 10.106/j.optom.2015.10.004

[41] Pauk SV, Petriček I, Jukić T, Popović-Suić S, Tomić M, Kalauz M, et al. Noninvasive tear film break-up time assessment using handheld lipid layer examination instrument. Acta Clin Croat. 2019;58:63-71. DOI: 10.20471/acc.2019.58.01.09

[42] Li N, Deng X, He M. Comparison of the Schirmer I test with and without topical anesthesia for diagnosis dry eye. Int J Ophthalmol 2012;5(4):478-481. DOI: 10.3980/j.issn.2222-3959.2012.04.14

[43] Clinch TE, Benedetto DA, Felberg NT, Laibson PR. Schirmer's test: A closer look. Arch Ophthalmol. 1983;101:1383-1386. DOI: 10.1001/archopht.1983.01040020385009

[44] Senchyna M, Wax MB. Quantitative assessment of tear production: A review of methods and utility in dry eye drug discovery. J Ocul Biol Dis Inform. 2008;1:1-6. DOI: 10.1007/s12177-008-9006-2

[45] Ibrahim OMA, Dogru M, Ward SK, Matsumo Y, Wakamatsu TH, Ishida K, et al. The efficacy, sensitivity, and specificty of strip meniscometry in conjunction with tear function tests in the assessment of tear meniscus. Invest Ophthalmol Vis Sci. 2011;52:2194-2198. DOI: 10.1167/iovs.10-5986

[46] Wright JC, Meger GE. A review of the Schirmer test for tear production. Arch Ophthalmol. 1962;67:564-565. DOI: 10.1001/archopht.1962.00960020564008

[47] Jones LT. The lacrimal secretory system and its treatment. Am J Ophthalmol. 1966;62(1):47-60. DOI: 10.1016/0002-9394(66)91676-x

[48] [No author listed]. Methodologies to diagnose and monitor dry eye disease: Report of the definition and classification subcommittee of the international dry eye workshop (2007). Ocul Surf. 2007;5(2):108-152. DOI: 10.1016/s1542-0124(12)70083-6

[49] Wood SD, Mian SI. Diagnostic tools for dry eye disease. European Ophthalmic Review 2016;10(2):101-107. DOI: 10.17925/EOR.2016.10.02.101

[50] Makateb A, Torabifard H. Dry eye signs and symptoms in night-time workers. J Curr Ophthalmol. 2017;29(4):270-273. DOI: 10.106/j.joco.2017.05.003

[51] Sakamoto R, Bennet ES, Henry VA, Paragina S, Narumi T, Izumi Y, et al. The phenol red thread tear test: A cross-cultural study. Invest Ophth Vis Sci. 1993; 34:3510-3513.

[52] Saleh TA, McDermott B, Bates AK, Ewings P. Phenol red thread test vs Schirmer's test: A comparative study. Eye 2006;20:913-915. DOI: 10.1038/sj.eye.6702052

[53] Tomlinson A, Blades KJ, Pearce EI. What does the phenol red thread test actually measure?. Optometry and Vision Science 2001;78(3):142-146.

[54] Vashisht S, Singh S. Evaluation of phenol red thread test versus Schirmer test in dry eyes: A comparative study. Int J Appl Basic Med Res. 2011;1(1):40-42. DOI: 10.4103/2229-516X.81979

[55] Baudouin C, Brignole F, Becquet F, Pisella P, Gogue A. Flow cytometry in impression cytology specimens. Invest Ophth Vis Sci. 1997;38(7):1458-1464.

[56] Singh R, Joseph A, Umapathy T, Tint NL, Dua HS. Impression cytology of the ocular surface. Br J Ophthalmol. 2005;89:1655-1659. DOI: 10.1136/bjo.2005.073916

[57] Baoudoin C. Nonroutine tests for dry eye disease. In: Asbell PA, Lemp MA, editors. Dry Eye Disease: The Clinician's Guide to Diagnosis and Treatment. New York: Thieme; 2006. p. 47-62. DOI: 10.1055/b-002-51025

[58] Lemp MA, Bron AJ, Baoudouin C, del Castillo JMB, Geffen D, Tauber J, et al. Tear osmolarity in the diagnosis and management of dry eye disease. Am J Ophthalmol. 2010;151(5):792-798. DOI: 10.1016/j.ajo.2010.10.032

[59] Schargus M, Wolf F, Tony HP, Meyer-ter-Vehn T, Geerling G. Correlaion between tear film osmolarity, dry eye disease, and rheumatoid arthritis. Cornea 2014; 33:1258-1261. DOI: 10.1097/ico.0000000000000257

[60] Masmali AM, Purslow C, Murphy PJ. The tear ferning test: A simple clinical technique to evaluate the ocular tear film. Clin Exp Optom. 2014;97:399-406. DOI: 10.1111/cxo.12160

Chapter 2

The Physiology of Tear Film

Abraham Kayal

Abstract

The precorneal tear film is a thin layer, about 2–5.5 μm thick, which overlays the corneal and conjunctival epithelium. It functions to lubricate and protect the corneal and eyelid interface from environmental and immunological factors as well as provide an optical medium. The tear film is depicted as a three-layered structure: lipid, aqueous, and mucous layers. Within each layer possesses a different composition which dictates its function. In common between the three layers are their homeostatic process of evaporation and drainage. Any dysfunction in either of the layers can result in Dry Eye Syndrome (DES). The composition, regulation, and pathology of tear film will be discussed in this chapter.

Keywords: Physiology, tear film, meibomian glands, lacriminal glands, conjunctival goblet cells, blink reflex

1. Introduction

The precorneal tear film is traditionally described as a structure made of three layers which make up a thickness of 2–5.5 μm [1]. The thickness of the tear film was a controversial topic, with many attempts to measure the full thickness through different imaging modalities. However, recent publications such as the DEWS II Tear Film state that ultrahigh resolution Optical Coherence Tomography (OCT) has recently resolved the debate over the tear film thickness. Furthermore, the tear film is now regarded as a complex blended two-layer structure comprising of an outer lipid layer and an inner muco-aqueous layer [1, 2]. However, to better understand the precorneal tear film, the traditional approach will be taken in this review. The three tear film layers serve to not only protect and provide nutrition to the cornea, but also act as the first refractive surface for light entering the eye. Of the three layers, the largest is the middle aqueous. (e.g. **Table 1**).

2. The layers of tear film

Traditionally, the tear film has been described as a three-layered structure composed of the deep mucinous, middle aqueous, and superficial lipid layers (e.g. **Figure 1**). All three layers overlay the corneal and conjunctival epithelium, forming a full thickness of 2–5.5 μm [1]. Generally, the functions of the tear film are to lubricate the corneal and eyelid interface, form a protective covering and a smooth optical surface at the air-eye interface, and provide an antibacterial medium for the cornea and conjunctiva. The tear film also acts as the main oxygen supply to the corneal epithelium and functions as a temporary depository for instilling topical therapeutic drugs. (e.g. **Figure 1**).

	Origin	Composition	Function
Mucin Layer	• Corneal and Conjuctival epithelial cells (Glycocalyx) • Conjunctival goblet cells & Glands of Manz (Mucous)	• Glycoprotein • Mucin	• Converts corneal epithelium to a hydrophilic surface for aqueous to hydrate. • Decreases corneal surface tension.
Aqueous Layer	• Lacriminal glands • Corneal epithelial cells • Conjunctival epithelial cells	• Water • Oxygen • Lysozymes, Lactoferrin, Betalysin, Immunoglobins • VEGF • Electrolytes	• Barrier to infection • Flushes debris • Wound healing • Provides energy for corneal metabolism • Corneal hydration
Lipid Layer	• Meibomian glands	• Cholesterol esters • Waxes	• Delays evaporation • Lowers surface tension • Provides optically smooth surface

Table 1.
Overview of the origin, composition, and function of the tear film layers.

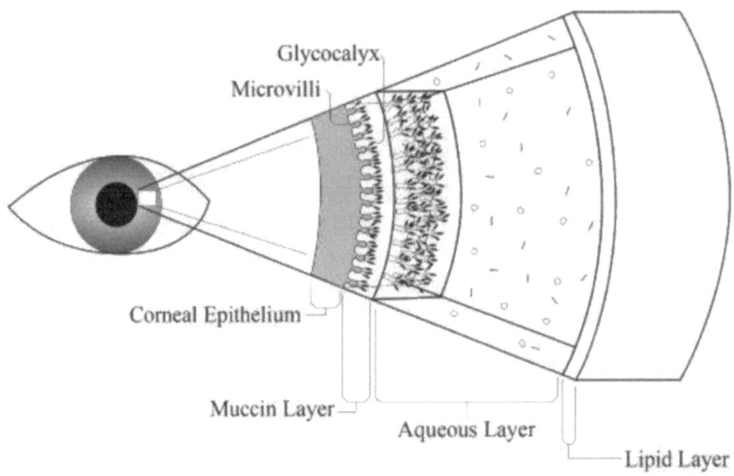

Figure 1.
Traditional 3-layered composition of tear film. Available via license: Creative commons attribution 4.0 international.

2.1 The mucinous layer

Most posteriorly sits the mucinous layer which has a thickness of 0.5 μm. It is composed of a mucin dominant gel formed by 2 layers: the glycocalyx and mucous layers. Posteriorly, the glycocalyx layer sits on the microvilli of the superficial corneal epithelium and is produced by the corneal and conjunctival epithelial cells [1, 2].

Overlying the glycocalyx layer is the mucous "blanket," a thick layer produced by the conjunctival goblet cells and the glands of Manz, lying in the crypts of Henle and in the bulbar conjunctiva, respectively [3]. This mucous layer is made of many gel-forming mucins and most significant of the mucin is MUC5-AC. Several studies

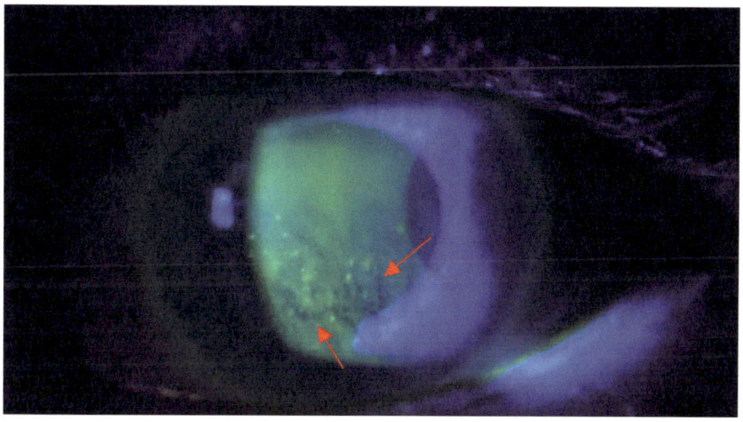

Figure 2.
TBUT with fluorescein dye tear break up (red arrow). Taken with permission from Kenny Chan [5].

have linked MUC5-AC decrease to DES. The function of the mucin is to transform the corneal surface into a hydrophilic surface [1, 2]. This transformation results in a reduction in corneal surface tension and provides the cornea with tear film stability, allowing the adhesion of the overlying aqueous layer, preventing the formation of dry spots. This decrease in surface tension also serves to lubricate and cushion the eye during all movements [3].

In order to test the integrity of the mucinous layer, the Tear Break-up Time (TBUT) test can be done. This test is used to assess for evaporative dry eye disease from the deficiency of mucin [4]. It is carried out by first instilling fluorescein into the patient's tear film. Afterwards, a cobalt blue illumination is shown onto the effected eye to observe the time elapsed between the last blink and the appearance of the first dry spot in the tear film (e.g. **Figure 2**). A TBUT of under 10 seconds is abnormal, indicating a problem with the mucinous layer's ability to form a hydrophilic layer [4].

Other abnormalities can occur which affect this layer include Vitamin A deficiency, Ocular Cicatricial Pemphigoid, Stevens-Johnsons Syndrome, and Alkali burns [6]. All mentioned conditions lead to the destruction of goblet cells with consequent loss of mucin production. As a result, a rapid breakdown of tear film occurs, even with adequate volume of aqueous layer.

2.2 The aqueous layer

The middle aqueous layer forms the largest part of the tear film thickness, at 2–6 μm [1]. Its main functions are to supply oxygen to the corneal epithelium, provide a protective layer against bacteria, and provide a healing media through VEGF. The aqueous layer is produced by the secretions of the lacriminal gland apparatus and its accessory glands. The aqueous layer can be secreted via reflex secretions or via its basal source. The reflex secretions are secreted by the main lacriminal gland whereas the basal source of the aqueous is secreted from the accessory lacriminal glands of Krause and Wolfring [7].

Unlike the mucinous layer, the release of aqueous is mediated by various methods: the autonomic nervous system, hormones, and psychological factors. The autonomic nervous system activates the lacriminal reflex through the sensory innervations at the corneal and conjunctival unmyelinated C-type fibers which form the subepithelial plexus at the superficial cornea [8]. The stimulation of the sensory nerves causes the parasympathetic system to increase the aqueous secretion and vasodilate the blood vessels supplying the lacriminal gland. Although the sympathetic nervous system plays a role in tear lacriminal aqueous secretion, the parasympathetic system predominates this reflex [8].

Androgens also play a role in the mediation of aqueous secretion from the lacriminal gland. Reduced serum androgen levels in women with altered endocrine states, such as women after menopause, ovariectomy, and during oral contraceptive use have been observed to have primary lacriminal deficiency, despite their variable estrogen levels. However, men who take anti-androgen therapy do not show signs of any change to tear secretion, suggesting that the androgen effect of the lacriminal gland may be sex specific [8]. Moreover, emotional expression also controls the secretion of aqueous from the lacriminal gland. The exact mechanism is currently unknown, and further research is needed to understand the neurobiology of human emotional crying [2, 8].

The aqueous layer is composed of 98% water, with the remaining 2% made up of Sodium, Potassium (6x that of plasma), Chloride, Bicarbonate, Calcium, Amino Acids, Oxygen, and VEGF (**Table 2**) [7]. The proteins found in the aqueous layer plays a significant role, as it supplies the cornea with a rich source of bactericidal enzymes. High in number of lysozymes, lactoferrin, betalysin, and immunoglobins, the aqueous layer provides a barrier to infection for the eye. The Immunoglobins, mostly IgA, are derived from the lymphoid tissue in the lacriminal gland stroma. Furthermore, the VEGF found in the aqueous provides the cornea with a source for healing [7, 9].

Due to the cornea's requirements to achieve transparency, there is no blood supply within its structure. Nevertheless, oxygen is needed for the corneal epithelium's aerobic metabolism. This oxygen is derived mainly from the aqueous layer of the tear film when the eyes are open and minorly from the conjunctival blood vessels when the eyes are closed. When the eyes are open, the tear film possesses a saturation of 155 mmHg of Oxygen which makes up 70% of ATP production at the corneal epithelium. The last 30% occurs when the eyes are closed, with the saturation of oxygen from the conjunctival blood vessels being 55 mmHg. If the individual is a contact lens wearer, the pO2 drops to around 15 mmHg when eyes are closed [9, 10]. Moreover, the aqueous layer smooths irregularities in the corneal surface providing an optical function.

To test the caliber of the aqueous layer, the Schirmer test can be performed. The Schirmer test is done using a special filter paper which is 5 mm wide and 35 mm long with the bent end placed between the palpebral conjunctiva of the lower eyelid and the bulbar conjunctiva of the eye. The eye is then closed for 5 minutes and the absorption of the fluid into the filter paper is measured in millimeters. The test can be done with or without the use of anesthetics (e.g. **Figure 3**) [11]. To evaluate the baseline secretions of the lacriminal gland, the test is done using anaesthestics, whereas the evaluation of reflex secretions along with baseline secretions is done without the use of anaesthestics. An individual with normal aqueous tear

Sodium	134–170 mmol/l
Potassium	20–40 mmol/l
Chloride	130 mmol/l
Bicarbonate	26 mmol/l
Calcium	0.61 mmol/l
Amino Acids	50 mg/l
Urea	4–7 mmol/l

Table 2.
Electrolytes and proteins making up 2% of aqueous [7].

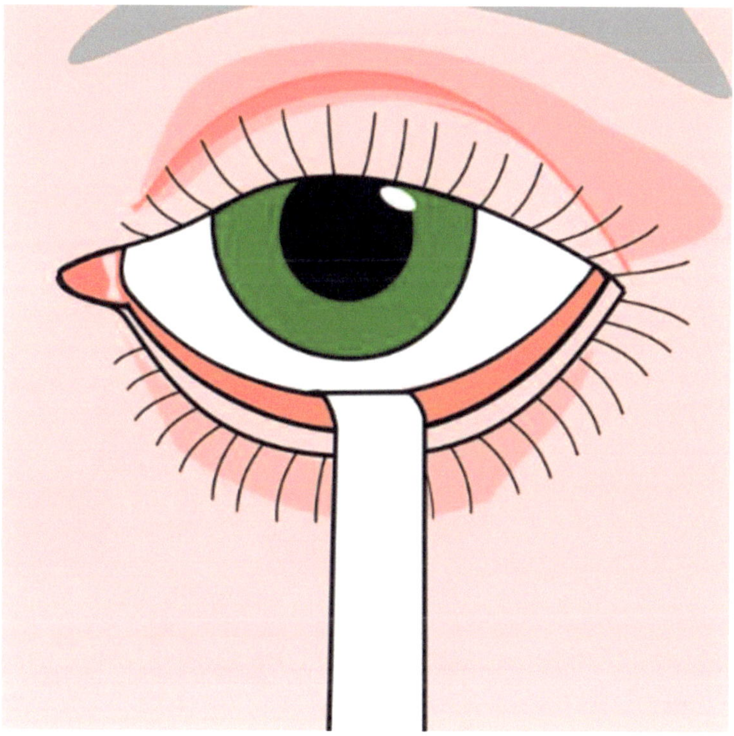

Figure 3.
Schirmer test. Available via license: Creative commons attribution-share alike 3.0 Unported.

production will have a reading of >15 mm after 5 minutes. Mild–moderate reduction of aqueous production is a reading from 5 to 14 mm after 5 minutes, and severe dryness is a reading of less than 5 mm [11, 12].

A deficiency of the aqueous layer is responsible for about 20% of cases of DES [11]. Such deficiency can be a result of advanced age, Sjogrens syndrome, Keratoconjunctivitis Sicca, familial dysautonomia, and side-effects of common ocular surgeries such as LASIK, PRK, and phacoemulsification [13, 14].

2.3 The lipid layer

The lipid layer is the most significant layer in terms of DES. Alterations of its thickness and composition are associated with DES. The lipid layer is the outermost layer of the precorneal tear film and is the thinnest at 0.04 μm. The lipids within this layer are secreted from mainly the meibomian glands, with minor contribution from the Moll and Zeiss glands located in the eyelids [1, 13, 15].

The lipid layer is composed of mostly cholesteryl esters and waxes, with the rest of its composition made up of diesters, fatty acids, cholesterol, and triacylglycerol. The main function of this layer is to prevent the rapid evaporation of tears, followed by the prevention of spillage of tears at the lid margin [16, 17]. This prevention is achieved by the formation of a water-tight seal with the closure of the lids. Furthermore, the lipid layer functions as a clear optical medium.

Deficiency of the lipid layer occurs with meibomian gland dysfunction (MGD). Of cases of dry eye, MGD makes up 60% of cases of DES [13]. With the dysfunction of the meibomian gland, the thickness of the lipid layer is decreased, leading to rapid evaporation of tears and spillage of tear film over the lid margin, ending in eye dryness. To individuals with DES, this spillage can give the false sensation

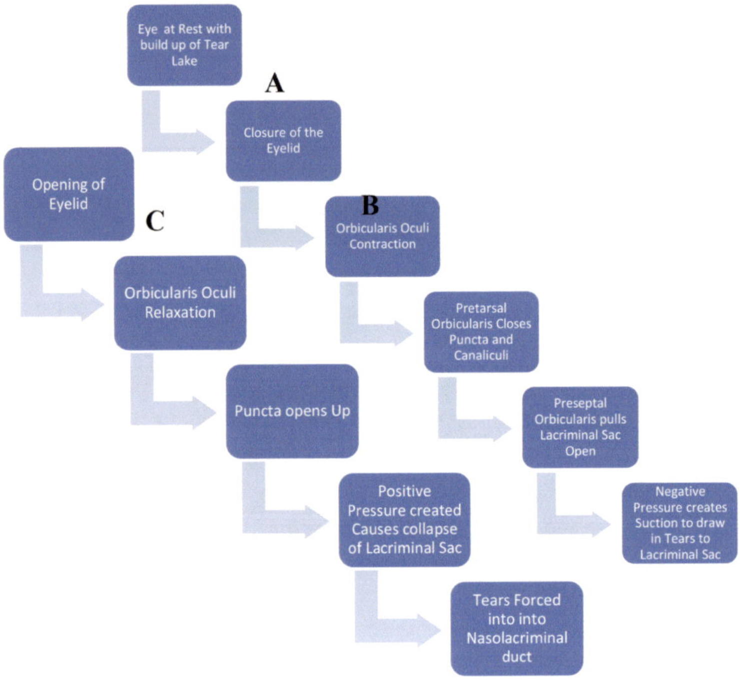

Figure 4.
Lacrimal pump mechanism corresponding with ***Figure*** *5.*

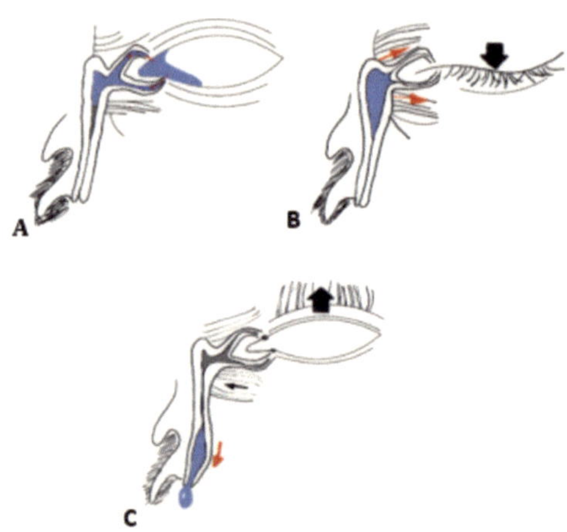

Figure 5.
Illustration of Lacrimal pump. (A) Pump at resting state. (B) Closure of eyelid. (C) Opening of eyelid.

of excessive watering as opposed to dryness. Other conditions effecting the meibomian glands are infections from *Staphylococcus aureus* and other bacteria which produce cholesterol esterase and fatty wax esterase capable of hydrolyzing the meibomian lipids and forming "froths" at the lid margin [18].

Non-invasive tests including interferometry, meibography, and meibometry are carried out to detect abnormalities in the lipid layer and meibomian gland. However, meibometry is the only test which measures the basal lipid production volume of the meibomian glands [17, 19, 20]. The test is done with the use of an 8-mm wide loop of translucent plastic tape and a "Laser Meibometer" which measures the optical density of the tape. Before beginning the test, the optical density of the plastic tape is measured with the laser meibometer as a control. While the patient is gazing upwards with their lower lid pulled downwards, the loop is then pushed against the lid margin with a pressure of 0 mmHg for 3 seconds and is set aside for 3 minutes to evaporate any tear fluid contaminants. Afterwards, the laser meibometer is used to measure the "casual" or basal lipid level. This measurement is calculated as (C-B) where C is the casual reading and B is the reading from the untouched tape [20].

3. Balance of tear film

The dynamics of the precorneal tear film are balanced through drainage and evaporation. The drainage of the tear film is regulated by neural reflexes, as opposed to evaporation which depends on the blink rate, temperature, humidity, and air velocity [21].

The drainage of the tear film is maintained by the lacriminal portion of the orbicularis muscle with blinking and is termed the "lacriminal pump mechanism" [22, 23]. This mechanism is controlled mainly by the closure and opening of the eyelids by the orbicularis oculi muscle, in turn effecting the pressure on the lacriminal sac as seen below (e.g. **Figures 3** and **4**):

4. Conclusion

The integrity of the tear film layer plays a significant role in the development of dry eye. Although extremely thin, the precorneal tear film holds a significant role in protecting the eye from environmental contamination and local or systemic pathology. Any alteration to the composition of each layer of tear film will drastically affect the function of that layer, and in turn compromise the health of the cornea.

Author details

Abraham Kayal
Institute of Ophthalmology, University College of London, London, United Kingdom

*Address all correspondence to: abraham.kayal@gmail.com

References

[1] Willcox MDP, Argüeso P, Georgiev GA, Holopainen JM, Laurie GW, Millar TJ, Papas EB, Rolland JP, Schmidt TA, Stahl U, Suarez T, Subbaraman LN, Uçakhan OO, MDk, Jones L; TFOS DEWS II Tear Film Report. Ocul Surf. 2017 July; 15(3): 366-403. doi:10.1016/j.jtos.2017.03.006

[2] Davidson HJ, Kuonen VJ. The tear film and ocular mucins. Vet Ophthalmol. 2004 Mar-Apr;7(2):71-7. doi: 10.1111/j.1463-5224.2004.00325.x. PMID: 14982585; PMCID: PMC7169288.

[3] TRB Chemedica International. The mucus layer. [Internet] 2016. Available from: https://vismed.trbchemedica.co.uk/business-professionals/understanding-the-tear-film/the-mucus-layer [Accessed 03-04-2021].

[4] University of Iowa. *Tear breakup time (TBUT)*. [Internet] 2021 Available from: https://webeye.ophth.uiowa.edu/eyeforum/atlas/pages/TBUT/index.htm [Accessed 14 April 2021].

[5] Kenny Chan, Tear Film Break Up Time, (2016) Available from: https://www.youtube.com/watch?v=p91NY_CuImY, (accessed: 27/04/2021)

[6] Hodges, Robin R, and Darlene A Dartt. "Tear film mucins: front line defenders of the ocular surface; comparison with airway and gastrointestinal tract mucins." Experimental eye research vol. 117 (2013): 62-78. doi:10.1016/j.exer.2013.07.027

[7] TRB Chemedica International. The acqueous layer. [Internet] 2016. Available from: https://vismed.trbchemedica.co.uk/business-professionals/understanding-the-tear-film/the-acqueous-layer [Accessed 03-04-2021].

[8] Dartt, Darlene A. "Neural regulation of lacrimal gland secretory processes: relevance in dry eye diseases." Progress in retinal and eye research vol. 28,3 (2009): 155-177. doi:10.1016/j.preteyeres.2009.04.003

[9] Neil J. Friedman, MD, Peter K. Kaiser, MD and William B. Trattler, MD. Review of Ophthalmology, 3rd Edition; 2018 p. 191. ISBN: 9780323390569

[10] National Research Council (US) Working Group on Contact Lens Use Under Adverse Conditions; Ebert Flattau P, editor. Considerations in Contact Lens Use Under Adverse Conditions: Proceedings of a Symposium. Washington (DC): National Academies Press (US); 1991. Environmental Gases and Contact Lens Wear. Available from: https://www.ncbi.nlm.nih.gov/books/NBK234120/

[11] Eyedocs. *Schirmer's Test*. [online] 2021 Available from: https://www.eyedocs.co.uk/ophthalmology-articles/cornea/505-schirmers-test [Accessed 01-04-2021].

[12] Brott NR, Ronquillo Y. Schirmer Test. [Updated 2020 Jun 9]. In: StatPearls [Internet]. Treasure Island (FL): StatPearls Publishing; 2021 Jan-. Available from: https://www.ncbi.nlm.nih.gov/books/NBK559159/

[13] Lukasz Cwiklik, Tear film lipid layer: A molecular level view, Biochimica et Biophysica Acta (BBA) - Biomembranes, Volume 1858, Issue 10,2016,Pages 2421-2430,ISSN 0005-2736, https://doi.org/10.1016/j.bbamem.2016.02.020.

[14] Finis D, Schrader S, Geerling G. Meibom-Drüsen-Dysfunktion [Meibomian gland dysfunction]. Klin Monbl Augenheilkd. 2012 May;229(5):506-13. German.

doi: 10.1055/s-0031-1299533. Epub 2012 May 16. PMID: 22592341.

[15] Kels BD, Grzybowski A, Grant-Kels JM. Human ocular anatomy. Clin Dermatol. 2015 Mar-Apr;33(2):140-146. doi: 10.1016/j.clindermatol.2014.10.006. PMID: 25704934.

[16] TRB Chemedica International. The lipid layer. [Internet] 2016. Available from: https://vismed.trbchemedica.co.uk/business-professionals/understanding-the-tear-film/the-lipid-layer [Accessed 04-04-2021].

[17] Bron AJ, Tiffany JM, Gouveia SM, Yokoi N, Voon LW. Functional aspects of the tear film lipid layer. Exp Eye Res. 2004 Mar;78(3):347-360. doi: 10.1016/j.exer.2003.09.019. PMID: 15106912.

[18] Poonam Mudgil; Antimicrobial Role of Human Meibomian Lipids at the Ocular Surface. Invest. Ophthalmol. Vis. Sci. 2014;55(11):7272-7277. doi: https://doi.org/10.1167/iovs.14-15512.

[19] Yokoi N, Komuro A. Non-invasive methods of assessing the tear film. Exp Eye Res. 2004 Mar;78(3):399-407. doi: 10.1016/j.exer.2003.09.020. PMID: 15106919.

[20] Wise, Ryan J et al. "Meibography: A review of techniques and technologies." Saudi journal of ophthalmology : official journal of the Saudi Ophthalmological Society vol. 26,4 (2012): 349-356. doi:10.1016/j.sjopt.2012.08.007

[21] Mathers W. Evaporation from the ocular surface. Exp Eye Res. 2004 Mar;78(3):389-394. doi: 10.1016/s0014-4835(03)00199-4. PMID: 15106917.

[22] Paulsen FP, Schaudig U, Thale AB. Drainage of tears: impact on the ocular surface and lacrimal system. Ocul Surf. 2003 Oct;1(4):180-191. doi: 10.1016/s1542-0124(12)70013-7. PMID: 17075649.

[23] Tear flow dynamics in the human nasolacrimal ducts--a pilot study using dynamic magnetic resonance imaging. Amrith S, Goh PS, Wang SC. Graefes Arch Clin Exp Ophthalmol. 2005 Feb;243(2):127-131.

Chapter 3

Lymphocytes in Dry Eye Disease

Alicia Vázquez-Mendoza, Danielle Vannan, Evelin G. Morales, Marisol I. González and José Luis Reyes Hernández

Abstract

The eye is a delicate organ that, along with other tissues such as the testicles and brain, is considered immune-privileged. Immune cells that reside in the eye must create a tolerogenic microenvironment to prevent unwanted aggressive inflammatory reactions that can compromise function. However, the eye is exposed to persistent environmental insult that may overwhelm immune tolerance and result in eye diseases from diverse origins (autoimmune, infectious, and inflammatory). The immune system plays a central role in the different phases of eye diseases, as alterations in immune cells in response to mechanical, chemical, or infectious stimuli initiate and amplify the immune response that lead to ocular tissue damage. Both resident and infiltrating immune cells also actively inhibit the immune response and promote tissue repair. Emerging evidence is leading to a better understanding of how and when lymphocytes, amongst other immune cells, contribute to inflammatory diseases such as dry eye disease (DED). We have compiled literature identifying the presence and participation of lymphocyte subpopulations that modulate DED from studies in both mice and humans. Notably, most mouse studies have relied on desiccant-stress-induced models (non-autoimmune DED), whereas human studies are predominantly in patients with Sjögren's syndrome (autoimmune DED).

Keywords: Dry eye disease, Lymphocytes, Inflammation, Ocular surface, Ocular therapy

1. Introduction

As a part of the central nervous system (CNS) and as an organ constantly exposed to a wide range of environmental stimuli, the eye has finely regulated immune-defense mechanisms. The eye can simultaneously respond to invading pathogens and tolerate beneficial, resident bacterial communities (ocular microbiota) while conducting its vital function, to capture luminous stimuli and transfer the signal to the brain so that they can be assimilated, and images are ultimately interpreted [1]. This finely tuned ocular function is protected by immune tolerance and defense mechanisms that are highly coordinated [2].

Physical barriers such as the blood–brain barrier (BBB) and the blood–retina barrier (BRB) prevent infiltration of systemic blood antigens into the eye protecting against a potential immune trigger [1]. Innate and adaptive immune cell populations are strategically positioned both dispersed throughout the ocular tissue and in organized follicles along the eye tissues (eye-associated lymphoid tissue (EALT)) [3]. This actively promotes a tolerogenic microenvironment, which is maintained by specific programs displayed by these immune cells. For example, antigen-presenting cells (APCs) express low levels of MHCII and costimulatory molecules (CD80 and CD86), and resident T cells show low production of interferon gamma (IFNγ) and enhanced transforming growth factor (TGF) β and interleukin 10 (IL-10). An additional, highly efficient eye component is tear production by the lacrimal gland. Tears are complex fluids whose role is to lubricate the ocular surface by binding to the epithelial surface via the inner mucin layer and to cooperate in microbial containment (both pathogen and commensals) as tears contain antimicrobial peptides (AMPs) such as lysozyme, lipocalin, lactoferrin, and immunoglobulin A (IgA), which inhibit microbial adherence [4–6]. Therefore, diverse surveillance pathways collaborate in a coordinated fashion to maintain eye homeostasis.

Despite the effort displayed by the above-mentioned tolerance and defense mechanisms, the eye faces challenging situations where overwhelming or persistent insults may ultimately alter homeostasis resulting in ocular pathologies. Eye disease can arise from the complex interaction between host (genetics, immunity, age, and sex) and the environment (air pollution, device exposure, and unsupervised medication). Multifactorial origins ranging from infectious and inflammatory to autoimmune can result in complex, yet unrelated co-morbidities.

1.1 Dry eye disease

Ocular surface inflammatory diseases such as dry eye disease (DED), which is currently the most frequent reason for ophthalmologic visits is projected to be an increasing eye morbidity due to lifestyle changes such as prolonged device use [7, 8]. DED is a group of diseases characterized by a strong inflammatory response targeting the ocular surface (conjunctiva, cornea, and meibomian and lacrimal glands) [7]. The most updated classification subdivides DED into two broad types: tear-deficient (aquodeficient) and evaporative DED. In the aquodeficient DED subtype, malfunctioning lacrimal glands (LGs) are often diagnosed. Deficiency in LG function is strongly associated with an autoimmune response targeting the body's salivary and lacrimal glands (Sjögren's syndrome) [7]. In evaporative DED, a reduced or altered lipidic composition of tear film is thought to be responsible [8]. Meibomian gland dysfunction (MGD) can result in decreased lipidic production, which is associated with infectious (bacterial and parasite) and non-infectious (hormones and duct obstruction) processes [7].

Manifestations compatible with those observed in DED are widely reported worldwide, positioning DED as the most common eye disease. DED is the most common eye pathology because this disease can emerge as a primary phenotype; that is, a local immune response is generated and sustained in the ocular surface and draining lymph nodes [9]. DED is also found as a secondary phenotype, where both autoinflammatory (e.g., colitis) [10, 11] and autoimmune diseases (Sjögren's syndrome, rheumatoid arthritis, and lupus) present DED symptoms [12–14]. The relevant finding that DED onset precedes autoimmune and non-autoimmune diseases in several patients is puzzling, and it has attracted interest from researchers worldwide, but the pathways remain to be elucidated.

Regardless of the origin, immune cells and their secreted products are the driving force of DED [9, 15]; therefore, a comprehensive understanding of the immune response as an initiator and perpetuating factor in DED is an area of intense research. Our immune system is composed of organs, cells, and molecules performing in a highly coordinated fashion; although finetuned mechanisms of regulation exist, pathologies prove that these mechanisms are not always limiting the intensity of the immune response. From the many cellular components of the immune response participating in DED, lymphocytes constitute one important component, which, when danger signals are detected, can be activated and become a disease-promoting player rather than homeostasis-maintaining cell type.

1.2 Lymphocyte diversity in the immune response

Lymphocytes are present in blood and lymph vessels and include innate and adaptive subtypes. All lymphocytes originate in the bone marrow (organ where all blood cells are created) from a common lymphoid precursor (CLP); however, not all lymphocytes reach mature status while in the bone marrow. For example, to achieve a mature T cell lineage, migration into the thymus is required, so they can complete their maturation through a complex process [16].

Classically, innate lymphocytes are represented by natural killer (NK) cells, whereas their adaptive counterparts include T and B cells. However, other lymphocytic subpopulations also exist in both innate and adaptive subtypes. The main difference between innate and adaptive lymphocytes is that the former express receptors encoded in the germline with limited diversity, such as toll-like receptors (TLRs) and carbohydrate-recognizing receptors (lectins), amongst others [17]. In contrast, adaptive lymphocytes express receptors generated by genetic recombination, which ultimately results in endless diversity. T and B lymphocytes perform gene rearrangements to express surface dimeric (two-chain, membrane-bound) T cell receptor (TCR) and B cell receptor (BCR), respectively. The TCR structure consists of alpha-beta chains, whereas the BCR structure is characterized by heavy and light chains forming a membrane-inserted immunoglobulin [18]. Thus, conventional innate lymphocytes are the NK cells and the conventional adaptive lymphocytes are the T and B cells.

An extended functional and phenotypical characterization of lymphocytes recently uncovered a growing diversity in lymphocytic subpopulations. A group of lymphocytes bearing low diversity TCRs and simultaneously expressing surface markers of NK was identified and named NKT cells [19]. Whereas most T cells express TCRs composed of classical alpha-beta chains, a less-abundant, mucosa-dwelling subtype of T cells express TCRs composed of gamma-delta chains, which is referred as $\gamma\delta$ T cells [20]. Currently, both NKT and $\gamma\delta$ T cells are considered unconventional T cells. More recently, other unconventional innate-like lymphocytes have been identified and these include the group 2 and group 3 innate lymphoid cells (ILC2s and ILC3s, respectively) [21] and mucosal-associated invariant T cells (MAITs), whose role has been widely explored in other mucosal surfaces (gut, skin, and lungs) [22].

B cells also have an innate-like counterpart; therefore, B cells are also subdivided into B1 and B2 cells. B1 cells mostly reside in the peritoneal and pleural cavity and produce low-affinity antibodies without stimulation (naturally produced antibodies), whereas B2 cells can produce high-affinity antibodies (affinity maturation process) and highly efficient memory responses [23].

Regarding their role within the immune response, all these lymphocytic cells contribute to a wide variety of both physiological and pathological processes. Lymphocytes residing and circulating during homeostatic conditions participate in immune surveillance; however, lymphocytes can be rapidly activated and collaborate in pathogen clearance. Furthermore, lymphocytes are involved in highly specialized functions such as the generation of memory responses, which allows increased intensity and efficiency in a secondary response. Lymphocytes additionally participate in the amplification of the immune response by rapidly releasing cytokines and chemokines (helper subpopulations) and preventing pathogen and tumor cells dissemination by elimination of infected or transformed cells (cytotoxic and killer types). Conversely, specific lymphocytes are also able to down-modulate the intensity of the immune response, thus turning these cells into regulatory subtypes, which are central in the resolution phase of the inflammatory process.

As above-mentioned, lymphocytes are active players both as promoters and regulators of inflammatory diseases. In the case of DED, how lymphocytes might be involved in the immunopathology of this disease was only recently described, and the understanding of these lymphocyte-driven pathological pathways may pave the way for new therapeutic opportunities.

2. The role of lymphocytes in DED

2.1 NK cells

NK cells are an early source of cytokines, such as interferon (IFN)γ and tumor necrosis factor (TNF)α and display cytotoxic features that place them in the first-line defense against intracellular pathogens and tumor cells. NK cells are grouped into the innate arm of the immune response since they lack antigen-specific receptors such as those found on adaptive cells (i.e., TCR and BCR) [24]. To fulfill their primary cytolytic role, NK cells are equipped with killer-activating receptors (KARs) as well as killer-inhibitory receptors (KIRs), whose role is integrating external signals that modulate the release of perforin and granzyme-containing granules that eliminate target cells. NK cells additionally express pattern-recognition receptors (PRRs), cytokine and chemokine receptors, and antibody Fc fragment receptors, all of which also contribute to NK functions [24].

NK cells were reported to be present in human conjunctiva samples obtained by cytology, and DED patients showed similar numbers of NK cells, suggesting that NK cell populations are not increased in DED [25]. Moreover, mouse studies showed that NK cells are found in the healthy conjunctiva, and DED induction caused a rapid infiltration of NK cells into the ocular surface (cornea and conjunctiva) as well as NK cell expansion in the draining cervical lymph node (CLN) [26–28]. A dual role for NK cells in the immunopathology of DED has been described. On one hand, it was reported that NK cells progressively decrease upon DED induction, which was paralleled by lower levels of IL-13 and goblet cell loss [29]. Thus, NK cells were identified as an IL-13 source. In turn, IL-13 prevented goblet cell loss, assigning a protective role to NK cells during DED (**Table 1**). Additionally, cyclosporine A (CsA) administration preserved NK cells and down-regulated pathogenic IFNγ and IL-17 cytokines [29]. On the other hand, a pathogenic role for NK cells in acute mouse DED was suggested since NK depletion with either antibodies (anti NK1.1) [26, 28] or antiasialo rabbit serum [27] ameliorated DED signs as gauged by less corneal damage (**Table 1**). Mechanistically, when IFNγ-producing NK cells were depleted, a reduced expression of costimulatory molecules (CD80 and CD86) in antigen-presenting cells (APCs), such as macrophages and dendritic cells (DCs), was found [26]. In line with this, immune neutralization of NK cells reduced CXCL9, CXCL10, and CXCL11 chemokines and IFNγ [28]. Furthermore, NK cells were identified as a source of the highly pathogenic cytokine IL-17 [27]. Ablation of NK cells resulted in matrix metalloproteinase (MMP) 3 and MMP9 attenuation in the cornea. Therefore, NK cell depletion strongly impacts pathogenic cytokine and chemokine output as well as APC activation, suggesting that rapid NK cell activation and further cytokine secretion in turn activate APCs to contribute to DED.

Mouse studies suggested that NK cells reside in the ocular surface and, upon DED induction, a highly dynamic cytokine response in these cells is initiated. However, depending on the cytokine profile released by NK cells, a differential impact on the DED outcome is observed. Altogether this mouse evidence suggested

Cell type	Strain	DED type/ model	Role disease	Ref
NK cells	Female C57BL6 Female and male C57BL/6 and STAT6 KO mice	Scopolamine-induced DED	NK cells were identified as an abundant source of IL-6, IL-17, IL-23, and IFNγ cytokines. NK cell depletion ameliorated DED outcome, related to decreased MMPs expression in cornea and lower costimulatory molecules on APC surface. A beneficial role was attributed to resident NK in maintaining Goblet cells by secreting IL-13.	[26, 29, 30]
NKT cells	Female and male C57BL/6 and STAT6 KO mice	Scopolamine-induced DED	NKT cells released IL-13, which collaborated in preserving goblet cells in the ocular surface.	[29]
ILCs	N.D.	N.D.	N.D.	
γδ T cells	Female C57BL/6 and male NOD mice	Scopolamine-induced DED	Upon DED induction, γδ T cell numbers tend to decrease on conjunctiva, suggesting a regulatory role on DED.	[30, 31]
T helper cells	Female C57BL/6	Scopolamine-induced DED	Th1 cells were present in draining lymph nodes from DED-induced mice and contributed to the recruitment of Th17 cells and inflammatory macrophages polarization. Th1 cells secreted IFNγ, which in turn induced goblet cell apoptosis and antagonized IL-13 effect on squamous epithelial cells.	[32, 33]
	Female C57BL/6 Female and male C57BL6, IFN-γKO Female BALB/c	Scopolamine-induced DED	Conjunctiva and cornea epithelia created a Th17 response. Memory Th17 cells promoted chronic DED. Th17 cells induced VEGF, which resulted in ocular angiogenesis. Th17 cells were highly pathogenic in DED, since they promoted MMPs expression and corneal barrier disruption, and suppressed the Treg response.	[34–38]
T cytotoxic cells	Female Lewis rats Female C57BL/6	Autoimmune DED Scopolamine-induced DED	Rats induced with autoimmune DED showed damaged lacrimal and salivary acinar cells, accompanied by a massive T cell infiltration, where $CD8^+$ T cells dominated over $CD4^+$ T cells. A pathogenic role for $CD8^+$ T cells was postulated. Upon acute DED induction, numbers of $CD8^+$ T cells were reduced in both conjunctival epithelium and stroma, and regulatory CD8+ T cells were described in DED.	[39–41]
Treg cells	Female BALB/c mice Female C57BL/6	Scopolamine-induced DED T cell transfer mediated-DED	$CD4^+CD25^+Foxp3^+$ T regs preserved tear production and reduced mononuclear cell and neutrophil infiltration when transferred into nude mice induced with Sjögren's syndrome-like disease. Treg cells from DED mice exhibited defective suppressive ability rather than decreased numbers.	[36, 39]

Cell type	Strain	DED type/ model	Role disease	Ref
B cells	Female and male C57BL/6	Scopolamine-induced DED	Plasma cells release IgG antibodies targeting components from the lacrimal gland (Kallikrein 13). When purified, these anti-kallikrein 13 antibodies induced DED signs. B cells could be activated more efficiently by IL-17 than by IFNγ. B cells infiltrated lacrimal glands in age-related DED.	[42–44]

Table 1.
The diverse roles of lymphocytes in rodent DED.

a dual role of NK cells in DED; a switch from normal protective IL-13-mediated to a pathogenic IFNγ- and IL-17-mediated role has been proposed for the eye-resident NK population [27]. What triggers either a protective or pathogenic program in NK cells and the role of NK cells in human DED remains to be determined.

2.2 NKT cells

NKT cells are a subgroup of innate-like lymphocytes that recognize lipid antigens presented by MHC class-I-like molecule (CD1d) and are identified by the co-expression of TCR and the NK-related NK1.1 marker. NKT cells are further divided into type I NKT or invariant NKT cells (iNKT) and type II NKT cells. Type I NKT cells express a semi-invariant TCR, whereas type II NKT cells possess a more diverse TCR repertoire. Upon NKT activation by either lipid antigens or bacterial products sensed by TLRs, these cells rapidly secrete large amounts of cytokines, such as IFN-γ, TNF-α, IL-2, IL-4, IL-5, and IL-13, which modulate the function of neighbouring innate and adaptive cells. In organs such as the liver, NKT cells are abundant and the main players of the local response; however, in the eye, NKT cells are shown to be a relevant cell type [45].

Pioneer studies identified NKT cells as the resident population in the mouse ocular surface. Cells isolated through immunobeads from the mouse ocular surface under homeostatic conditions were identified using reliable NKT markers (TCR and NK1.1). Moreover, these cells were found to be an important source of IL-13; through the secretion of this molecule, NKT cells help to preserve the goblet cells, which promote ocular surface stability by producing mucins (**Table 1**) [29]. The same group of researchers subsequently confirmed their findings by identifying cells positively stained for CD3 and NK1.1 markers, a phenotype compatible with NKT cells in conjunctiva samples from healthy mice [30]. Interestingly, these authors reported that the actual number of NKT cells was higher than the number of conventional T cells (CD4 and CD8 lymphocytes), suggesting that, like in other epithelial tissues, NKT cells are abundant in the ocular surface [30].

Therefore, the evidence, although minimal but convincing, shows that NKT cells are fundamental for maintenance of the ocular surface through communication with goblet cells. Impaired crosstalk between these cells adds to the development of DED, so a protective role can therefore be inferred for NKT cells in DED.

2.3 γδ T cells

T lymphocytes bearing a TCR composed of gamma-delta chains (γδ T cells) are less abundant than αβ T cells; however, γδ T cells represent a major T cell population in the epithelial tissues such as the skin, and gastrointestinal and reproductive tracts. As part of the intraepithelial lymphocytes (IELs), γδ T cells are central players in the protection and homeostasis of surfaces in constant contact with the external environment. Specifically in the eye, γδ T cells collaborate in maintaining ocular immune privilege [46].

Early evidence arose from studies on the non-diabetic obese (NOD) mouse strain, which, upon ageing, develop a Sjögren's-syndrome-like disease. When DED was induced in NOD mice via scopolamine delivery, symptoms such as a decreased tear volume and goblet cell density as well as increased corneal permeability were observed (**Table 1**). The authors noted a significant decline in the numbers of γδ T cells in the conjunctival epithelium during the acute phase of DED [31]. Intriguingly, using the same DED model (scopolamine administration) in a different mouse strain (C57BL/6), decreased numbers of γδ T cells present in the conjunctival epithelium were observed when DED was induced, but increased γδ T cells were visible in flow cytometry samples [30]. Moreover, a strain-dependent effect of γδ T cells on tear volume was found where C57Bl/10 J (B10) mice lacking γδ T cells presented higher tear volume compared with C57BL/6 J (B6) similarly lacking γδ T cells [47].

Regarding human DED, the role of γδ T cells has not yet been explored; however, Sjögren's syndrome patients are reported to present altered numbers of γδ T cells. One may speculate that as DED is frequently observed in Sjögren's syndrome patients, in human DED secondary to autoimmune disease, a modified γδ T cell response is expected.

Salient evidence suggests that the depletion of γδ T cells is a hallmark of experimental DED, supporting an immunoregulatory role of the γδ T cells despite them being a well-known source of pathogenic IL-17 (**Table 1**). This regulatory role is further supported by mice lacking γδ T cells not developing anterior-chamber-associated immune deviation (ACAID), and corneal grafts are more tolerated when γδ T cells are present [48]. An anti-inflammatory role for γδ T cells in DED is currently accepted.

2.4 T helper cells

T cells and B cells compose the lymphocytes of the adaptive immune system. T cells are further subdivided into T helper (Th) and T cytotoxic (Tc) groups, identified as $CD4^+$ and $CD8^+$, respectively. $CD4^+$ Th cells are abundant lymphocytes with the primary role of secreting cytokines to amplify the immune response by promoting crosstalk amongst cells. Once activated, Th cells proliferate and polarize, which means they selectively secrete specific groups of cytokines and chemokines. Currently, effector Th cells are grouped based on the cytokines released as follows: Th1 cells secrete IFNγ; Th2 cells secrete IL-4, IL-5, and IL-13; Th17 cells secrete IL-17; and Th22 cells secrete IL-22. Compared with effector Th cells, regulatory Th cells produce IL-10 and are termed type 1 T regulatory cells (Tr1). As Th cells have been shown to be highly pathogenic and contribute to inflammatory disease, specifically Th1 and Th17 cells, these subpopulations are under intense research in DED.

$CD4^+$ and $CD8^+$ T cells are less abundant on the healthy ocular surface compared to γδ T cells and it has been noted that $CD4^+$ T cells outnumber $CD8^+$ T cells. Induction of DED in rodents and in patient with DED, T cells are found to consistently infiltrate the ocular surface. In early mouse studies of DED, upon desiccant-stress-induced DED, increasing numbers of CD4+ T cells were observed in the cornea, conjunctiva, and lacrimal gland tissues [39] (**Table 1**). It was demonstrated that transferring these cells is enough to induce DED in mice lacking T and B cells, showing that $CD4^+$ T cells are largely responsible for inducing DED (**Table 1**) [39]. Additional reports also provided evidence of $CD4^+$ T cells driving autoimmune DED in autoimmune regulator-knockout (Aire KO) mice [49] and being present in lacrimal glands in a novel autoimmune model of DED in rats [40]. This same population was found to be expanded within draining lymph nodes from DED-induced mice [32]. Similarly, human studies showed that DED patients with an autoimmune origin (Sjögren's syndrome) and with a non-autoimmune origin (non-Sjögren) presented comparable numbers of $CD4^+$ T cells assessed per immunohistochemistry using conjunctival samples [50].

Research has also focused on identifying specific subtypes of $CD4^+$ T cells involved in DED, where Th1 and Th17 cells have received the most attention since DED induction was found to cause increased transcripts of both IFNγ and IL-17 in the ocular surface [34]. Expansion of IFNγ-secreting $CD4^+$ T cells co-expressing CXCR3 and CCR5 chemokine receptors (Th1 polarized T cells) in the regional lymph nodes (submandibular and cervical) has been reported [32, 51]. Interestingly, IFNγ may be highly relevant at the onset of DED, but its role during chronic DED may be limited [49]. The relevance of Th1 in DED immunopathology can be inferred due to the detrimental effect of IFNγ on the ocular surface, since the presence of IFNγ receptor was demonstrated on the conjunctival and corneal epithelium [33]. Additionally, IFNγ is amongst the cytokines elevated in tears from DED patients and was shown to alter mucin secretion by inducing cell death in conjunctiva-residing goblet cells [52]. A diminished density of goblet cells resulting from IFNγ administration was also reported [41]. IFNγ was also found to be responsible for inducing apoptosis in lacrimal gland cells [53].

Once polarized and activated, Th2 cells secrete IL-4, IL-5, and IL-13 cytokines. Even though DED is a Th1-prone inflammatory condition, it has been reported that tear samples from DED patients contain elevated levels of IL-4, IL-5, and IL-13, suggesting activation of the Th2 pathway [54–56]. Intriguingly, Th2 cytokines were detected elevated in tears from DED-induced experimental animals [57]; however, the contribution of the cytokines to mouse DED appears to be strain-dependent, since DED induction caused different cytokine and chemokine profiles in C57BL/6 compared with BALB/c mice [58]. Although IL-13 has been shown to prevent goblet cell loss, innate lymphocytes (NK and NKT cells) were demonstrated to be the cellular source; thus, we can speculate that Th2 cells collaborate in preserving mucin-producing cells as well. However, this remains to be proven.

In terms of Th17 cells, DED induction creates a Th17-inducing microenvironment as gauged by a rapid increase in IL-6 and IL-23 expression. Th17 cells have been readily detected in draining lymph nodes from acute and chronic DED-induced mice [34, 35], and their pathogenic role is supported by experimental evidence showing that IL-17 neutralization attenuated corneal damage. Furthermore, Th17 cells emerging in experimental DED were shown to be resistant to suppression exerted by T regulatory cells and, unlike Th1 cells, Th17 cells survived longer periods of time, adding to chronic DED [36]. A wide variety of negative effects on the ocular surface have been attributed to Th17 cells and IL-17 including promotion of MMPs expression, corneal barrier damage, and induction of angiogenesis via vascular endothelial growth factor (VEGF) (**Table 1**) [37].

Another group of $CD4^+$ T cells addressed in the context of DED is the T regulatory (Treg) subtype. Treg cells are identified by the expression of the transcription factor Foxp3 and high levels of CD25 and can suppress cell proliferation. Niederkorn et al. demonstrated that the presence of $Foxp3^+$ Tregs prevented DED symptoms induced by the adoptive transfer of ocular-surface-specific T effector cells (**Table 1**) [39]. Thereafter, it was shown that a percentage of lymph node residing $Foxp3^+$ Tregs remains unaltered upon DED induction but their suppressive ability is reduced compared with their counterparts from non-DED animals, when tested *in vitro* [36]. Recently, administration of histone deacetylase inhibitors (HDACi)-containing microspheres that stabilized $Foxp3^+$ expression reduced DED signs [59].

Several CD4⁺ T subtypes have been identified in DED, and the roles of Th1, Th17 and Tregs have been highlighted. A well-established pathogenic role of Th1 and Th17 in inducing ocular surface damage through the release of IFNγ and IL-17, respectively, has been assigned. In sharp contrast, Treg cells are responsible for restraining exacerbated inflammatory responses in the ocular surface. Therefore, the balance between these CD4⁺ T cells subpopulations seems to be determinant for the onset and chronicity of DED.

2.5 T cytotoxic cells

Although T cytotoxic cells (CD8⁺ T cells) also contribute by producing cytokines such as IFNγ, they are best known for their cytolytic functions. CD8⁺ T cells contain granules with perforin and granzyme, which are delivered to the target cells with the goal of inducing cell death via membrane damage and cellular content release. A few studies have addressed the role of CD8⁺ T cells in DED, and the evidence is controversial. It was suggested that CD8⁺ T cells might play a regulatory role, since a significant loss of CD8⁺ T cells in the conjunctiva was found to accompany the development of DED [30] and DED patients showed increased CD4/CD8 compared with healthy donors (**Table 2**) [25]. Furthermore, thrombospondin 1 (TSP1)-deficient mice exhibited DED symptoms accompanied by dramatic lacrimal gland cell infiltration, where CD4⁺ T cells were significantly increased; CD8⁺ T cells were not increased compared with those in mice expressing TSP1 [65]. Conversely, CD8⁺ T cells were the dominant cell type in severely damaged ducts within lacrimal glands of rats induced with an autoimmune DED model [40]. In line with this,

Cell type	DED type	Role in Disease	Ref
NK cells	Non SS	A putative limited role was assumed since NK numbers were not different between healthy controls and DED patients	[25]
NKT cells	N.D.	N.D.	
ILCs	N.D.	N.D.	
γδ T cells	N.D.	N.D.	
T helper cells	SS and Non SS	Highly infiltrated in lacrimal glands from SS patients. Increase in CD4⁺ T cells numbers correlated with dryness, hyperemia, and itching score. Th cells secreted IL-21, which in turn favors B cell transition to plasma cells. Different T cell subpopulations were associated with differential DED signs, for instance, CD4⁺CCR7⁺CD45RO⁻CD45RA⁺ correlated with hyperemia, whereas patients with CD4⁺CCR7⁻CD45RO⁺CD45RA⁻CD69⁻CD103⁻ cells showed reduced tear film break up time (BUT). Memory T cells (CD4⁺CD45RA⁻) correlated with corneal damage and serum Ro antibodies.	[60–64]
T cytotoxic cells	SS and Non SS	The presence of Tc cells with the phenotype CD8⁺CCR7⁺CD45RO⁻CD45RA⁺ positively correlated with hyperemia. Conversely, CD8⁺CCR7⁻CD45RO and CD45RA⁺CD69⁺CD103⁺ were abundant when patients largely exhibited reduced tear film	[63]
B cells	SS untreated	Produced antinuclear antibody (ANA)	[62]

SS; Sjögren's Syndrome, N.D.; not documented.

Table 2.
The role of lymphocytes in human DED.

using a mouse autoimmune model of Sjögren's syndrome, lacrimal glands presented a massive infiltration of $CD8^+$ T cells [53], and aged mice displaying ocular surface pathology (corneal irregularity and conjunctival goblet cell loss) presented increased numbers of $CD8^+$ T cells [42].

Therefore, additional studies are needed to better understand the role of $CD8^+$ T cells during DED development. In the current literature, most of the mouse studies investigate immunological changes during the acute stage of disease; however, it is well-known that DED is a chronic disease. Thus, the role of resident cells might contribute to the infiltration of additional pathogenic populations responsible for perpetuating the inflammatory process. A differential role of $CD8^+$ T cells occurring during early versus late stages of disease cannot be ruled out.

2.6 B cells

B lymphocytes complement T cells in adaptive immunity and in generating immune memory responses. B cells perform a variety of functions in homeostatic conditions and following the initiation of an adaptive immune response. These functions include cytokine release, antigen processing and presentation, and their signature role as antibody-producing cells. In mucosal surface immunosurveillance, the presence of IgA is pivotal in limiting pathogen invasion. In the EALT, B cells are present in both diffuse and organized (follicles) forms to support their function. B cells are essential in eye-associated immune responses ranging from surveillance to autoimmune-mediated diseases and allergies.

As mentioned above, human DED can arise from autoimmune diseases (Sjögren's syndrome and rheumatic) and DED was proposed to be a mucosal autoimmune disease [66]. Despite being proposed as an autoimmune disease, the role of B cells in both human and mouse DED has not been completely addressed.

In terms of studies in patients with Sjögren's syndrome, autoimmune-response-targeting exocrine glands (salivary and lacrimal) are the driving force of the disease; however, human studies mostly focused on the salivary glands rather than lacrimal glands and the ocular surface. Information learned from patients with Sjögren's syndrome linking B cell subpopulations and eye manifestations is still lacking. More thorough research on B cells and their participation during mouse DED must be conducted.

Thus far, the role of B cells in mouse models of DED may be model-dependent. When DED was induced via pharmacological inhibition of the lacrimal gland function (desiccant stress), no significant changes were observed regarding the percentage of B cells present in the tissue (**Table 1**) [30]. Likewise, the NOD autoimmune model of DED was attenuated by blocking high-mobility group box 1 (HMGB1) with neutralizing antibodies; however, no substantial changes in either the percent of B cells or in IL-10-producing B cells were found [67]. Conversely, when DED symptoms were evaluated in aged mice, without any additional chemical agent, B cell numbers were found to be increased accompanying DED development [42]. A pathogenic role of B cells in DED is supported by the findings showing that a DED-like disease can be generated by transferring antibody-containing serum (purified IgG isotype) obtained from mice previously induced with DED for three weeks [43]. The transfer of antibodies required the presence of complement proteins to cause ocular surface damage [43], suggesting that in eye tissue exposed to desiccant stress, antibodies targeting lacrimal gland components like kallikerin 13 are induced (**Table 1**). Additionally, IL-17 collaborates in B cell proliferation and plasma cells generation [44].

Recent findings show that B cells are instrumental in DED, either human or mouse; however, the only mechanism through which these B cells induce eye damage is proposed to be by secreting antibodies targeting lacrimal gland antigens.

To prove that additional pathways are also regulated by B cells resulting in Sjögren-associated and non-Sjögren-related DED, future studies are required.

3. The future players in DED

Both novel techniques (single cell sequencing and massive flow cytometry) and the discovery of novel functions have allowed the better characterization of immune cell populations, revealing a wider diversity of lymphocyte subpopulations than previously thought. As an example, mucosal-residing ILCs have emerged as central early regulators in the immune response. In the case of inflammatory diseases, including DED, lymphocyte populations have specifically received more attention than others, which does not imply that the populations that we do not yet understand are less important. Notably, MAITs and ILCs are only beginning to arise as potential drivers in eye pathologies. Few studies have, for instance, shown that extremely low numbers of ILC2s reside in the mouse cornea and are recruited upon corneal epithelial injury, where they are required for cornea tissue repair [68]. Additional studies described that cells, presumably ILCs, can be isolated from human and mouse conjunctiva [69]. In eye pathologies, MAITs were reported to be increased in acute anterior uveitis [70] and ILCs played no role in ocular infection with herpes simplex virus (HSV)2 [71]. Thus, a role for MAITs and ILCs cannot be ruled out in DED, and future evidence will further our understanding of the expanding universe of lymphocytes in DED.

4. Targeting lymphocytes as therapy for DED

The findings summarized here strongly indicate that resident lymphocytes can rapidly be activated when the microenvironment in the ocular surface is altered by the lack of tears (aquodeficient) or have altered composition (evaporative). Evidence now suggests that innate and adaptive lymphocytes regulate the onset and persistence of DED. For instance, NK are shown to switch their cytokine response, which is critical for initiating DED, whereas other innate lymphocytes such as γδ T cells and NKT cells are mostly suppressive in homeostasis, and DED may parallel the loss of these populations. Regarding the adaptive lymphocytes, T and B populations are responsible for promoting chronicity. The important role of lymphocytes during DED is also supported using diverse therapeutics aimed to attenuate lymphocyte activation; thus, controlling lymphocyte populations has long been considered an efficient therapy for DED. These strategies include diverse methods of controlling T cells response; for instance, cyclosporine A (CsA) eyedrops targeted cell proliferation [72, 73]. It has been reported that commercially available CsA formulations such as Restasis (0.05% CsA, Allergan) and Ikervis (0.1% CsA, Santen) are highly effective in treating DED, however, side effects which are thought to be vehicle-related, have been reported [74, 75]. Therefore, improving CsA delivery is the current challenge. Recently, results from phase II and phase III clinical trials have been released. Wirta *et al.* published their results from a USA-centered phase II trial (efficacy, safety and tolerability) using a water- and oil-free emulsion containing a 0.1% CsA dose termed CyclASol for 16 weeks that resulted in earlier and more effective relief in adult DED patients compared to Restasis (Allergan) administered under the same protocol [76]. In an independent study, CsA was encapsulated in nanomicelles to enhance its effectiveness. The authors hypothesized that given the hydrophobic nature of CsA that dampens aqueous solubility encapsulating CsA in nanomicelles would help to solubilize CsA and ultimately increase its efficacy.

The 0.09% CsA nanomicellar solution, termed OTX-101, was administered for 84 days in individuals (18–90 years old) and significantly increased integrity of the ocular surface [77]. Thus, CsA still remains as one of the most recommended DED therapies and these efforts to enhance its effects by using novel ways of delivery with promising results keep expectations high to achieve complete DED remission.

Additional DED therapies targeting lymphocytes include eyedrops containing anti-CD4 antibodies suppressing cell activation [78] and more recently, blocking T cell infiltration by antagonizing LFA1 (Lifitegrast) [79]. Therapies increasing regulatory lymphocytes are another method of ameliorating DED. Rebamipide, which promotes the expansion of regulatory adaptive lymphocytes, yielded promising results in autoimmune DED [80]. More sophisticated agents such as histone deacetylase inhibitor (HDACi)-containing microspheres aimed at stabilizing regulatory T cells have also shown beneficial effects on DED symptoms [59].

Thus, currently approved drugs as well as experimental evidence (NK depletion) show that regulating both innate and adaptive lymphocytes can be a complimentary therapy for strategies to restore healthy tears. The more we understand about how lymphocytes participate in DED, the greater the possibilities of mitigating DED.

5. Conclusion

There has been a tremendous breakthrough concerning DED research, from previously being considered only as a syndrome to what is now recognized as the most common eye pathology. Experimental models have been instrumental for the better understanding of DED immunopathology; unfortunately, human studies are underrepresented. Convincing evidence obtained mostly from animal studies shows that lymphocytes have important implications in DED, placing Th1, Th17, and B cells as the main pathological subtypes, which seem to be in constant competition with immune cell populations mostly displaying regulatory features such as Tregs that are ultimately responsible for lessening the intensity of disease-promoting counterparts. Contrary to the extensive work that has been done describing how adaptive cells are active players in both promoting and regulating DED, evidence is just starting to uncover surprising roles attributed to innate and innate-like lymphocytes. As we have reviewed here, strong evidence, up to now, suggests possible "program switching" in resident innate cell populations like NKs whereas other cells such as NKT and T cells rather display a regulatory role contributing to a tolerogenic microenvironment on the ocular surface. More recently, cell populations like ILCs have been described expanding upon eye tissues injury, which paves the way to uncover novel roles for these ILCs in a variety of eye pathologies, similarly to other organs. Continued research will help to clarify how these populations contribute to DED immunopathology. It is evident that additional human studies would complement and validate these findings, with the ultimate goal of identifying new therapeutic targets based on modulating lymphocyte responses. We have also shown that some of the most effective DED treatments indeed target lymphocyte populations (cyclosporine A and LFA-1 inhibitors) and current trials are aimed to develop a more efficacious way to deliver these drugs with proved benefit in DED therapy.

Acknowledgements

J.L.R. is funded by the programa de apoyo a proyectos de investigación e innovación tecnológica (PAPIIT,) project number IN224520. A.V.M. is funded by PAPIIT, project number IN226220.

Author details

Alicia Vázquez-Mendoza[1], Danielle Vannan[2], Evelin G. Morales[3], Marisol I. González[3] and José Luis Reyes Hernández[3]*

1 Laboratory of Ocular Inflammatory Diseases, College of Optometry, Faculty of Higher Studies Iztacala, UNAM, Tlalnepantla de Baz, Estado de México, Mexico

2 Boston Scientific Corporation, Endoscopy Division, Marlborough, MA, USA

3 Laboratory of Experimental Immunology and Immune-Regulation of the Gut Liver Axis, Faculty of Higher Studies Iztacala, Unit of Biomedicine (UBIMED), UNAM, Tlalnepantla de Baz, Estado de México, Mexico

*Address all correspondence to: jlreyes@iztacala.unam.mx

References

[1] Kels, B.D., A. Grzybowski, and J.M. Grant-Kels, *Human ocular anatomy.* Clin Dermatol, 2015. **33**(2): p. 140-6.

[2] Knop, E. and N. Knop, *Anatomy and immunology of the ocular surface.* Chem Immunol Allergy, 2007. **92**: p. 36-49.

[3] Knop, E. and N. Knop, *[Eye-associated lymphoid tissue (EALT) is continuously spread throughout the ocular surface from the lacrimal gland to the lacrimal drainage system].* Ophthalmologe, 2003. **100**(11): p. 929-42.

[4] Tiffany, J.M., *The normal tear film.* Dev Ophthalmol, 2008. **41**: p. 1-20.

[5] Zhou, L., et al., *In-depth analysis of the human tear proteome.* J Proteomics, 2012. **75**(13): p. 3877-85.

[6] Knop, E., N. Knop, and P. Claus, *Local production of secretory IgA in the eye-associated lymphoid tissue (EALT) of the normal human ocular surface.* Invest Ophthalmol Vis Sci, 2008. **49**(6): p. 2322-9.

[7] Willcox, M.D.P., et al., *TFOS DEWS II Tear Film Report.* Ocul Surf, 2017. **15**(3): p. 366-403.

[8] Johnson, M.E. and P.J. Murphy, *Changes in the tear film and ocular surface from dry eye syndrome.* Prog Retin Eye Res, 2004. **23**(4): p. 449-74.

[9] Knop, N. and E. Knop, *Regulation of the inflammatory component in chronic dry eye disease by the eye-associated lymphoid tissue (EALT).* Dev Ophthalmol, 2010. **45**: p. 23-39.

[10] Cury, D.B. and A.C. Moss, *Ocular manifestations in a community-based cohort of patients with inflammatory bowel disease.* Inflamm Bowel Dis, 2010. **16**(8): p. 1393-6.

[11] Czompa, L., et al., *Corneal Manifestations of Inflammatory Bowel Disease.* Semin Ophthalmol, 2019. **34**(7-8): p. 543-550.

[12] Vehof, J., et al., *Advances, limitations and future perspectives in the diagnosis and management of dry eye in Sjogren's syndrome.* Clin Exp Rheumatol, 2020. **38 Suppl 126**(4): p. 301-309.

[13] Kemeny-Beke, A. and P. Szodoray, *Ocular manifestations of rheumatic diseases.* Int Ophthalmol, 2020. **40**(2): p. 503-510.

[14] Read, R.W., *Clinical mini-review: systemic lupus erythematosus and the eye.* Ocul Immunol Inflamm, 2004. **12**(2): p. 87-99.

[15] Clayton, J.A., *Dry Eye.* N Engl J Med, 2018. **378**(23): p. 2212-2223.

[16] Koch, U. and F. Radtke, *Mechanisms of T cell development and transformation.* Annu Rev Cell Dev Biol, 2011. **27**: p. 539-62.

[17] Janeway, C.A., Jr. and R. Medzhitov, *Innate immune recognition.* Annu Rev Immunol, 2002. **20**: p. 197-216.

[18] Nielsen, S.C.A. and S.D. Boyd, *Human adaptive immune receptor repertoire analysis-Past, present, and future.* Immunol Rev, 2018. **284**(1): p. 9-23.

[19] Makino, Y., et al., *Predominant expression of invariant V alpha 14+ TCR alpha chain in NK1.1+ T cell populations.* Int Immunol, 1995. 7(7): p. 1157-61.

[20] Nielsen, M.M., D.A. Witherden, and W.L. Havran, *gammadelta T cells in homeostasis and host defence of epithelial barrier tissues.* Nat Rev Immunol, 2017. **17**(12): p. 733-745.

[21] Vivier, E., et al., *Innate Lymphoid Cells: 10 Years On.* Cell, 2018. **174**(5): p. 1054-1066.

[22] Pellicci, D.G., H.F. Koay, and S.P. Berzins, *Thymic development of unconventional T cells: how NKT cells, MAIT cells and gammadelta T cells emerge.* Nat Rev Immunol, 2020. **20**(12): p. 756-770.

[23] Wang, Y., et al., *B Cell Development and Maturation.* Adv Exp Med Biol, 2020. **1254**: p. 1-22.

[24] Sivori, S., et al., *Human NK cells: surface receptors, inhibitory checkpoints, and translational applications.* Cell Mol Immunol, 2019. **16**(5): p. 430-441.

[25] Barabino, S., et al., *Immune response in the conjunctival epithelium of patients with dry eye.* Exp Eye Res, 2010. **91**(4): p. 524-9.

[26] Chen, Y., et al., *Interferon-gamma-secreting NK cells promote induction of dry eye disease.* J Leukoc Biol, 2011. **89**(6): p. 965-72.

[27] Ren, G., et al., *Association of killer cell immunoglobulin-like receptor and human leukocyte antigen-C genotype with dry eye disease in a Chinese Han population.* Genet Test Mol Biomarkers, 2012. **16**(8): p. 910-4.

[28] Coursey, T.G., et al., *Desiccating stress-induced chemokine expression in the epithelium is dependent on upregulation of NKG2D/RAE-1 and release of IFN-gamma in experimental dry eye.* J Immunol, 2014. **193**(10): p. 5264-72.

[29] De Paiva, C.S., et al., *Homeostatic control of conjunctival mucosal goblet cells by NKT-derived IL-13.* Mucosal Immunol, 2011. **4**(4): p. 397-408.

[30] Zhang, X., et al., *NK cells promote Th-17 mediated corneal barrier disruption in dry eye.* PLoS One, 2012. **7**(5): p. e36822.

[31] Yoon, K.C., et al., *Desiccating environmental stress exacerbates autoimmune lacrimal keratoconjunctivitis in non-obese diabetic mice.* J Autoimmun, 2008. **30**(4): p. 212-21.

[32] El Annan, J., et al., *Characterization of effector T cells in dry eye disease.* Invest Ophthalmol Vis Sci, 2009. **50**(8): p. 3802-7.

[33] Pflugfelder, S.C., R.M. Corrales, and C.S. de Paiva, *T helper cytokines in dry eye disease.* Exp Eye Res, 2013. **117**: p. 118-25.

[34] Chen, Y., et al., *Chronic dry eye disease is principally mediated by effector memory Th17 cells.* Mucosal Immunol, 2014. **7**(1): p. 38-45.

[35] Chauhan, S.K. and *R. dana*, *Role of Th17 cells in the immunopathogenesis of dry eye disease.* Mucosal Immunol, 2009. **2**(4): p. 375-6.

[36] Chauhan, S.K., et al., *Autoimmunity in dry eye is due to resistance of Th17 to Treg suppression.* J Immunol, 2009. **182**(3): p. 1247-52.

[37] Chauhan, S.K., et al., *A novel pro-lymphangiogenic function for Th17/IL-17.* Blood, 2011. **118**(17): p. 4630-4.

[38] De Paiva, C.S., et al., *IL-17 disrupts corneal barrier following desiccating stress.* Mucosal Immunol, 2009. **2**(3): p. 243-53.

[39] Niederkorn, J.Y., et al., *Desiccating stress induces T cell-mediated Sjogren's Syndrome-like lacrimal keratoconjunctivitis.* J Immunol, 2006. **176**(7): p. 3950-7.

[40] Jiang, G., et al., *A new model of experimental autoimmune keratoconjunctivitis sicca (KCS) induced in Lewis rat by the autoantigen Klk1b22.*

Invest Ophthalmol Vis Sci, 2009. **50**(5): p. 2245-54.

[41] De Paiva, C.S., et al., *Dry eye-induced conjunctival epithelial squamous metaplasia is modulated by interferon-gamma.* Invest Ophthalmol Vis Sci, 2007. **48**(6): p. 2553-60.

[42] McClellan, A.J., et al., *Ocular surface disease and dacryoadenitis in aging C57BL/6 mice.* Am J Pathol, 2014. **184**(3): p. 631-43.

[43] Stern, M.E., et al., *Autoantibodies contribute to the immunopathogenesis of experimental dry eye disease.* Invest Ophthalmol Vis Sci, 2012. **53**(4): p. 2062-75.

[44] Subbarayal, B., et al., *IL-17 Augments B Cell Activation in Ocular Surface Autoimmunity.* J Immunol, 2016. **197**(9): p. 3464-3470.

[45] Zhu, S., H. Zhang, and L. Bai, *NKT cells in liver diseases.* Front Med, 2018. **12**(3): p. 249-261.

[46] Skelsey, M.E., J. Mellon, and J.Y. Niederkorn, *Gamma delta T cells are needed for ocular immune privilege and corneal graft survival.* J Immunol, 2001. **166**(7): p. 4327-33.

[47] O'Brien, R.L., et al., *alphabeta TCR(+) T cells, but not B cells, promote autoimmune keratitis in b10 mice lacking gammadelta T cells.* Invest Ophthalmol Vis Sci, 2012. **53**(1): p. 301-8.

[48] Xu, Y. and J.A. Kapp, *gammadelta T cells are critical for the induction of anterior chamber-associated immune deviation.* Immunology, 2001. **104**(2): p. 142-8.

[49] Chen, Y.T., et al., *Pax6 downregulation mediates abnormal lineage commitment of the ocular surface epithelium in aqueous-deficient dry eye disease.* PLoS One, 2013. **8**(10): p. e77286.

[50] Stern, M.E., et al., *Conjunctival T-cell subpopulations in Sjogren's and non-Sjogren's patients with dry eye.* Invest Ophthalmol Vis Sci, 2002. **43**(8): p. 2609-14.

[51] Yoon, K.C., et al., *Expression of CXCL9, -10, -11, and CXCR3 in the tear film and ocular surface of patients with dry eye syndrome.* Invest Ophthalmol Vis Sci, 2010. **51**(2): p. 643-50.

[52] Zhang, X., et al., *Interferon-gamma exacerbates dry eye-induced apoptosis in conjunctiva through dual apoptotic pathways.* Invest Ophthalmol Vis Sci, 2011. **52**(9): p. 6279-85.

[53] Bian, F., et al., *Altered balance of interleukin-13/interferon-gamma contributes to lacrimal gland destruction and secretory dysfunction in CD25 knockout model of Sjogren's syndrome.* Arthritis Res Ther, 2015. **17**: p. 53.

[54] Enriquez-de-Salamanca, A., et al., *Tear cytokine and chemokine analysis and clinical correlations in evaporative-type dry eye disease.* Mol Vis, 2010. **16**: p. 862-73.

[55] LaFrance, M.W., L.E. Kehinde, and R.J. Fullard, *Multiple cytokine analysis in human tears: an optimized procedure for cytometric bead-based assay.* Curr Eye Res, 2008. **33**(7): p. 525-44.

[56] Lam, H., et al., *Tear cytokine profiles in dysfunctional tear syndrome.* Am J Ophthalmol, 2009. **147**(2): p. 198-205 e1.

[57] Corrales, R.M., et al., *Strain-related cytokine profiles on the murine ocular surface in response to desiccating stress.* Cornea, 2007. **26**(5): p. 579-84.

[58] Yoon, K.C., et al., *Expression of Th-1 chemokines and chemokine receptors on the ocular surface of C57BL/6 mice: effects of desiccating stress.* Invest Ophthalmol Vis Sci, 2007. **48**(6): p. 2561-9.

[59] Ratay, M.L., et al., *Controlled release of an HDAC inhibitor for reduction of*

inflammation in dry eye disease. Acta Biomater, 2018. **71**: p. 261-270.

[60] Reinoso, R., et al., *Differential cell proliferation, apoptosis, and immune response in healthy and evaporative-type dry eye conjunctival epithelia.* Invest Ophthalmol Vis Sci, 2011. **52**(7): p. 4819-28.

[61] Choi, W., et al., *Expression of CCR5 and its ligands CCL3, -4, and -5 in the tear film and ocular surface of patients with dry eye disease.* Curr Eye Res, 2012. **37**(1): p. 12-7.

[62] Jin, L., et al., *CD4+CXCR5+ follicular helper T cells in salivary gland promote B cells maturation in patients with primary Sjogren's syndrome.* Int J Clin Exp Pathol, 2014. 7(5): p. 1988-96.

[63] Bose, T., et al., *Tissue resident memory T cells in the human conjunctiva and immune signatures in human dry eye disease.* Sci Rep, 2017. 7: p. 45312.

[64] Joachims, M.L., et al., *Sjogren's Syndrome Minor Salivary Gland CD4(+) Memory T Cells Associate with Glandular Disease Features and have a Germinal Center T Follicular Helper Transcriptional Profile.* J Clin Med, 2020. **9**(7).

[65] Turpie, B., et al., *Sjogren's syndrome-like ocular surface disease in thrombospondin-1 deficient mice.* Am J Pathol, 2009. **175**(3): p. 1136-47.

[66] Stern, M.E., C.S. Schaumburg, and S.C. Pflugfelder, *Dry eye as a mucosal autoimmune disease.* Int Rev Immunol, 2013. **32**(1): p. 19-41.

[67] Kim, K.H., et al., *Effects of subconjunctival administration of anti-high mobility group box 1 on dry eye in a mouse model of Sjgren's syndrome.* PLoS One, 2017. **12**(8): p. e0183678.

[68] Liu, J., et al., *Local Group 2 Innate Lymphoid Cells Promote Corneal Regeneration after Epithelial Abrasion.* Am J Pathol, 2017. **187**(6): p. 1313-1326.

[69] Yoon, C.H., et al., *Distribution of Interleukin-22-secreting Immune Cells in Conjunctival Associated Lymphoid Tissue.* Korean J Ophthalmol, 2018. **32**(2): p. 147-153.

[70] Huang, J.C., et al., *Preliminary Report on Interleukin-22, GM-CSF, and IL-17F in the Pathogenesis of Acute Anterior Uveitis.* Ocul Immunol Inflamm, 2019: p. 1-8.

[71] Hirose, S., et al., *Roles of Type 1, 2, and 3 Innate Lymphoid Cells in Herpes Simplex Virus 1 Infection In Vitro and In Vivo.* J Virol, 2019. **93**(13).

[72] de Paiva, C.S., et al., *Topical cyclosporine A therapy for dry eye syndrome.* Cochrane Database Syst Rev, 2019. **9**: p. CD010051.

[73] Kunert, K.S., et al., *Analysis of topical cyclosporine treatment of patients with dry eye syndrome: effect on conjunctival lymphocytes.* Arch Ophthalmol, 2000. **118**(11): p. 1489-96.

[74] Sall, K., et al., *Two multicenter, randomized studies of the efficacy and safety of cyclosporine ophthalmic emulsion in moderate to severe dry eye disease. CsA Phase 3 Study Group.* Ophthalmology, 2000. **107**(4): p. 631-9.

[75] Leonardi, A., et al., *Efficacy and safety of 0.1% ciclosporin A cationic emulsion in dry eye disease: a pooled analysis of two double-masked, randomised, vehicle-controlled phase III clinical studies.* Br J Ophthalmol, 2019. **103**(1): p. 125-131.

[76] Wirta, D.L., et al., *A Clinical Phase II Study to Assess Efficacy, Safety, and Tolerability of Waterfree Cyclosporine Formulation for Treatment of Dry Eye Disease.* Ophthalmology, 2019. **126**(6): p. 792-800.

[77] Goldberg, D.F., et al., *A Phase 3, Randomized, Double-Masked Study of OTX-101 Ophthalmic Solution 0.09% in the Treatment of Dry Eye Disease.* Ophthalmology, 2019. **126**(9): p. 1230-1237.

[78] Hayashi, Y., et al., *Effective treatment of a mouse model of Sjogren's syndrome with eyedrop administration of anti-CD4 monoclonal antibody.* Arthritis Rheum, 2004. **50**(9): p. 2903-10.

[79] Holland, E.J., et al., *Lifitegrast for the Treatment of Dry Eye Disease: Results of a Phase III, Randomized, Double-Masked, Placebo-Controlled Trial (OPUS-3).* Ophthalmology, 2017. **124**(1): p. 53-60.

[80] Fu, R., et al., *Rebamipide ophthalmic solution modulates the ratio of T helper cell 17/regulatory T cells in dry eye disease mice.* Mol Med Rep, 2019. **19**(5): p. 4011-4018.

Chapter 4

Diagnosis of Dry Eye

Shrinkhal, Rupal Verma and Anupam Singh

Abstract

Dry eye is a multifactorial disease and hence single test cannot diagnose dry eye. Diagnosis of dry eye needs careful assessment of the symptoms along with battery of investigations. Many questionnaires have been developed to assess the symptoms of dry eye disease (DED). Some of the important questionnaires are Ocular Surface Disease Index (OSDI), Dry Eye Questionnaire (DEQ-5), Impact of Dry Eye on Everyday Living (IDEEL), National Eye Institute's Visual Function Questionnaire (NEI VFQ-25) and Dry Eye-Related Quality-of-Life Score (DEQS). Investigations for dry eye mainly target on the tear secretion, tear clearance, tear volume, tear film stability, tear evaporation, ocular surface damage, lipid layer of the tear film, chemical properties of the tear film and inflammation of the ocular surface. There are many investigations that target on the above parameters and helps in accurate diagnosis of Dry eye disease (DED).

Keywords: Dry eye disease, Ocular surface index (OSDI), Schirmers test, Phenol red test, Fluorescein

1. Introduction

1.1 Definition

Tear Film and Ocular Surface Society (TFOS) Dry Eye Workshop (DEW) II amended the definition of dry eye into "Dry eye is a multifactorial disease of the ocular surface characterized by a loss of homeostasis of the tear film, and accompanied by ocular symptoms, in which tear film instability and hyperosmolarity, ocular surface inflammation and damage, and neurosensory abnormalities play etiological roles" [1]. So, basically patients are not required to present with a particular set of symptoms to be diagnosed as dry eye disease (DED) but rather homeostasis of the tear film is more emphasized upon.

1.2 Classification

DED is classified into two main categories by TFOS DEW II. The two main types are the following-

1. Aqueous deficiency – It occurs due to deficient tear production.

2. Evaporative – Meibomian gland disease (MGD) lead to deficiency of lipid layer which ultimately leads to excessive evaporation of tears [1].

The diagnosis of DED is not only based upon investigations but rather it depends on both the investigations and signs and symptoms of DED.

2. Questionnaires

Numerous questionnaires have been developed till date to study dry eye symptoms for many purposes such as diagnosis and quantification of DED, to study epidemiology of the disease, to assess effects of the treatment and its impact on the quality of life. The questionnaires are as follows-.

2.1 Ocular Surface Disease Index (OSDI)

It is a questionnaire consisting 12 questions, developed by the Outcome Research Group at Allergan which was designed for quick assessment of the symptoms of DED and their impact on vision related problems such as visual disturbance (poor vision or blurred vision) and visual function problems (difficulty in watching TV. working on a computer, driving at night and reading) [2].

The response to all the questions is graded on a scale of 0 to 4 -

a. none of the time

b. some of the time

c. half of the time

d. most of the time

e. all of the time

The following formula is then used to calculate the OSDI [3].

$$\text{OSDI} = \frac{(\textit{sum} \text{ of scores for } \textit{all} \text{ questions answered}) \times 100}{(\text{total number of questions answered}) \times 4} \tag{1}$$

A randomized study was performed on 68 patients admitted in ophthalmology Polyclinic of the Dumlupinar University from December 2005 to April 2006. Patients of 18 years and above were included in the study. The history taking and OSDI calculation was done by the same physician. Then after the routine ophthalmic assessment, the Schirmer test and TBUT were performed by another physician. The correlation analysis was done between Schirmer test, TBUT and OSDI scores. The patients were divided into 3 groups according to the OSDI scores and they are as follows-

- Group 1 had patients with low OSDI score of 0–20 points
- Group 2 had patients with moderate OSDI score of 21–45 points
- Group 3 had patients with high OSDI score of 46–100 points [3].

The result showed there was a statistically significant difference between TBUT test scores of patients with low and high OSDI scores ($p = .043$), there was no significant difference between Schirmer test scores of the three groups. They concluded that although there is no internationally accepted criterion for the diagnosis of DED as of now, the OSDI is a standardized questionnaire to evaluate symptoms, and can easily be performed and used to support the diagnosis of DED [3].

2.2 Dry Eye Questionnaire (DEQ-5)

It is a questionnaire in which 4 dimensions are used to measure a series of symptoms. The 4 dimensions are -.

a. Frequency of watery eyes.

b. Degree of bother.

c. Late day intensity of discomfort and dryness (PM intensity).

d. Morning intensity of discomfort and dryness (AM intensity).

DEQ-5 scores of ≥ 6 establish suspicion of DED and indicates further clinical testing and of ≥ 12 establishes a suspicion of Sjogren syndrome (SS) [4].

A study reported that 10% of patients with non-Sjogren syndrome DED and 30% of patients with Sjogren syndrome complained of impaired vision while few of the other studies reported that 42% and 80% of patients with Sjogren syndrome experienced impaired vision [5–7].

It is believed that open-eye conditions might affect symptom progression as visual problems generally increase in intensity over the day [8].

2.3 Impact of Dry Eye on Everyday Living (IDEEL)

The questionnaire has 2 items related to visual problems.

a. Blurry vision

b. Sensitivity to light, glare, and/or wind.

Statistically significant differences were observed between various patients od DED with varying level of severity and in responses to the IDEEL questionnaire scores [9].

2.4 National Eye Institute's Visual Function Questionnaire (NEI VFQ-25)

NEI VFQ-25 is a questionnaire that checks visual function by focusing on seven visual domains including general vision, near vision, distance vision, peripheral vision, color vision, driving difficulties and ocular pain. DED patients have poor NEI VFQ-25 scores for the subscales of general health, general vision, ocular pain, short distance vision activities, long distance vision activities, vision-related social function, vision-related mental health, vision-related role difficulties, vision-related dependency, and driving [10, 11].

2.5 Dry Eye-Related Quality-of-Life Score (DEQS)

This questionnaire developed in Japan. It has shown strong correlations with 4 subscales of the NEI VFQ-25 namely Ocular Pain, Near Vision, Distance Vision, and Mental Health [12].

2.6 Computer-vision symptom scale (CVSS17)

It is a Rasch linear scale containing 17 items. It explores 15 different symptoms of computer-related visual and ocular symptoms and is considered very valuable in computer related ocular morbidities. The CVSS17 includes a broad range of symptoms such as photophobia and excessive blinking [13].

2.7 McMonnies' Questionnaire (MQ)

It is a screening instruments for DED that reported sensitivity to be varying between 87–98% and specificity between 87% and 97% [14, 15]. It consists of 12 questions. Every question has polytomous response options that vary in number and type [16].

2.8 Ocular Comfort Index (OCI and OCI-C)

It was developed by Johnson and Murphy in 2007. It allows the quick assessment of the ocular comfort and grading the severity of DED. It uses Rasch analysis to produce estimates on a linear scale. It contains 15 items [17].

2.9 Symptoms Assessment in Dry Eye (SANDE)

It is based on 100 mm horizontal linear visual analog scale that quantifies both severity and frequency of dry eye symptoms. It consists of 2 questions [18].

2.10 Standard Patient Evaluation of Eye Dryness (SPEED)

It is based on both frequency and severity of the symptoms of the DED. It was designed to track diurnal and long-term symptom changes over a period of 3 months. The total score was calculated by adding the scores from both the frequency and severity parts of the questionnaire.

The symptoms inquired by the SPEED questionnaire include dryness or grittiness or scratchiness, soreness or irritation, burning sensation or watering and ocular fatigue reported and scored as sometimes – 1, often – 2 and constant – 3 and whether these symptoms pose no problems –0, were tolerable - 1, uncomfortable - 2, bothersome - 3, or intolerable –4 [19].

There are 3 more questionnaires which were developed to diagnose DED in the contact lens wearers –.

2.11 Contact Lens Dry Eye Questionnaire (CLDEQ)

It was developed by Begley [20]. It was used to investigate the frequency and severity of the symptoms of DED in contact lens wearers. It is quite similar to DEQ but the only difference is that patients here are using contact lens. It consists of 36 items [21]. It divides symptoms into nine subscales -

- Dryness

- Discomfort
- Visual impairment
- Irritation and soreness
- Grittiness or scratchiness
- Burning sensation
- Foreign body sensation
- Itching
- Photophobia

2.12 8-Item Contact Lens Dry Eye Questionnaire (CLDEQ-8)

The CLDEQ-8 is a short form of the CLDEQ questionnaire that was designed to describe symptoms among contact lens wearers [21].

2.13 Contact lens impact on Quality of life (CLIQ)

It is a questionnaire containing 28 items. It is based on Rasch analysis and shows good validity and reliability. Boer suggested that the psychometric properties of CLIQ were of high quality [22].

It is important to emphasize that these Questionnaires are not diagnostic tool, however can give a good clinical assessment of the problem. It acts as preliminary tool of assessment and is meant for screening purposes. Proper diagnosis requires a battery of additional tests. These above questionnaires act as adjunct to the clinical tests and cannot replace them in any form.

3. Diagnosis and ancillary testing

3.1 Aim

Investigations of DED are set with following goals -.

a. To confirm the clinical diagnosis of DED.

b. To quantify the DED.

Various tests have been devised to diagnose DED but no test can singly give you a diagnosis of DED. The correct way to diagnose DED it to correlate between the signs and symptoms of patients and the investigations planned.

3.2 Parameters to be measured

The following parameters are measured by tests to diagnose DED –.

a. Tear secretion.

b. Tear clearance.

c. Tear volume.

d. Tear film stability.

e. Tear evaporation.

f. Ocular surface damage.

g. Tear film chemical properties.

h. Lipid layer.

3.3 Investigations

3.3.1 To test the tear secretion and tear volume

3.3.1.1 Schirmer test

It is a test to quantify the tear production.

It is done with a blotting paper strip of 5 X 35 mm which is popularly known as Whatman filter paper number 41.

Method of application- It is folded 5 mm from the inner end which is rounded and placed in the lower fornix at the junction of middle and outer one-third and kept for 5 minutes. Touching the cornea or lashes should be avoided. Eyes should be gently closed during the procedures [23].

The normal tear production varies between 0.5 to 0.67 ml of tears/day and that wets more than 15 mm of the strip.

The Schirmer test are basically of 3 types but the most important amongst them are the first two.

- Schirmer's test I –It is done without the use of topical anesthesia and measures maximum basic plus reflex tear secretion.

- Schirmer's test II - It is done with the help of anesthesia. A drop of anesthesia is put in the eye, excess is wiped out with the help of filter paper. Then Whatman strip is placed same as in Schirmer test I. It measures only the basal tear secretion.

- Schirmer's test III - The patient is advised to look directly in the sun and it is done to know about the reflex tear secretion. It is dangerous and of no diagnostic value, so not used.

The cut-off values for diagnosis have been proposed as ≤5 mm/5 min to ≤10 mm/5 min with 77–85% sensitivity and 70–83% specificity [23].

This test lacks repeatability and shows variable results, so a single test should not be used to diagnosis rather a series of abnormal results in Schirmer's test raise a suspicion of DED. However, low cost of this test makes it one of the most commonly used tests clinically.

- Variations

3.3.1.1.1 Strip meniscometry

A variation of the above test is available now-a-days, which is done by dipping a strip into tear meniscus for 5 seconds. 25 mm polyethylene terephthalate is used to make the strip and it is covered with a urethane-based material [24]. The value ≤ 4 mm raises suspicion of DED. When used alone it has a sensitivity and specificity of 84% and 58% respectively and when combined with Tear film break-up time test the sensitivity is reduced to 81% but the specificity increases to 99% [25].

3.3.1.1.2 1-minute Schirmer test

It was proposed by Nelson to decrease the ocular discomfort and save time by decreasing the time of performing the test from 5 minutes to 1 minute [26]. The cut-off value was set to be 6 mm. Bawazeer and Hodge et al. in 2003 concluded that the 1-minute Schirmer test with anesthesia highly correlates with the 5-minute Schirmer test with anesthesia [27]. In cases of severe dry eye, a value of ≤ 5.5 mm in a 5-minute Schirmer test highly correlates with 2 mm in a 1-minute Schirmer test while in cases of mild to moderate dry eye a value of 5–10 mm in a 5- minute Schirmer test corresponds with 3–6 mm in a 1-minute Schirmer test.

3.3.1.2 Phenol red thread test (PRT)

It uses a thin cotton thread impregnated with pH-sensitive dye "phenol red". When the dye is dry, the thread is of yellow color, but when the dry is moistened by tears, the thread turns red (as the tears has slightly alkaline pH between 7 and 8) [28].

Method of application- the folded end of the thread is hooked over the lower eyelid margin in the temporal one-third if the eyelid for 15 seconds.

It has few advantages, as it is small in dimension so less chance of reflex tearing and the minimal amount of dye on thread decreases the chances of reflex tearing [29, 30]. It suggests that the reading of PRT is indirect and realistic measure of the tear volume in resting phase [31, 32]. But despite these potential advantages it is rarely used in clinical practice as it is manufactured only in few countries which makes their supply costly.

A cut-off value of 20 mm is used for differentiation of DED with and without aqueous deficiency [33]. Sensitivity and specificity of a cut-off value of 10 mm are 25% and 93% respectively [34].

Doughty et al. concluded that there is no statistically significant difference in the PRT performed with open or closed eyes [35].

3.3.2 To test the tear clearance

3.3.2.1 Fluorescein clearance test

Method- 5 μl of 2% fluorescein dye is instilled in the eyes. One set of Schirmer papers are inserted for each 10-minute interval for 30 minutes. The amount of strip becoming wet and the disappearance of the dye were recorded. Nasal stimulation is done using a cotton tip along with the last strip to induce reflex tear secretion.

It is used to measure basal tears, reflex tears and tear clearance all at the same time.

A cut-off value of ≥ 3 mm at the 10-minute interval suggests normal tear secretion. If the dye cannot be detected at the 20-minute interval, it is known as "Clearance" [36].

It has many advantages such as it is inexpensive, easy to perform, availability of the materials used is adequate. The disadvantages are same as in standard Schirmer test. Jordan and Baum et al. in 1980 reported that the above disadvantages cannot be suppressed by use of topical anesthesia [37].

3.3.2.2 Tear function index (TFI)

Method- The procedure is similar to the Schirmer test with anesthesia, but it uses 10-μl of 0.5% fluorescein.

Fluorescein is instilled into the lower conjunctival fornix and after 5 minutes of instillation the length of the wetted portion of the strip is measured and the intensity of the staining of dye is compared to the standard strips. The rate at which the color of the fluorescein dye fades is used to determine the tear clearance rate (TCR). It is graded as 1, 1/2, 1/4, 1/8, 1/16 1/32, 1/64, 1/128 and 1/256.

$$TFI = \frac{\text{Values of Schirmer test with anesthesia}}{TCR} \tag{2}$$

Kaye et al. proposed a variation of TFI by suggesting use of prepared strip containing 1.3 μl of 0.5% fluorescein. They reported that 10 μl of fluorescein use increases the volume of tear and it may also act as a stimulant. This in turn limits the applicability of the TFI test [38].

3.3.2.3 Fluorophotometry

Fluorophotometry is useful clinical tool, because an increased corneal uptake of fluorescein demonstrates subtle damage to the corneal epithelium. In humans, measurements of the penetration of fluorescein across the corneal epithelium can be used in diagnosing or monitoring dry eye disease. It is an excellent test but the need of the machine itself makes it a costly test so it not much used in clinical practice.

3.3.3 To test the tear volume

3.3.3.1 Tear meniscus assessment by Meniscometry

Tear meniscus height (TMH), curvature (TMR), and cross-sectional area (TMA) are used in clinical practice widely and have good accuracy rate and correlate well with other tests of DED [39, 40]. However, they are very much operated dependent. They have other drawbacks such as dependency on time from blink, fluorescein instillation. It can be influenced by the temperature, humidity, air velocity, illumination and location of measurement along the lid margin.

Now-a-days portable digital meniscometry with application software being installed in the iPod touch are being used. They have good reproducibility, good correlation with both the conventional video and Optical coherence tomography (OCT) meniscometry and it detects tear meniscus changed after the instillation of artificial tears.

At present, OCT meniscometry studies parameters such as upper and lower TMH, TMA, TMR and tear meniscus depth most commonly. Intra-observer and inter-observer repeatability are good with spectral-domain OCT meniscometry. All these measurements in the OCT meniscometry are machine dependent and can be influenced by the following conditions - conjunctivochalasis, LIPCOF, disorders of lid margin congruity, and apposition between the lid and ocular surface [41–44]. But it has many advantages such as it is non-invasive and image is taken rapidly and its simple but analysis of the image may take time [45]. It is an excellent but costly tool to test tear volume.

3.3.4 To test the tear film stability

3.3.4.1 Tear film break-up time (TBUT)

This is the time interval between the last complete blink and the appearance of the first randomly distributed dry spot [46, 47]. It is the most commonly done test for assessing the tear film stability.

It can either be done with or without fluorescein 2% dye. When done with dye it is known as Fluorescein break-up time (FBUT). The dye enhances the visibility of tear film but it also reduces the stability of the tear film and therefore the measurement may not be accurate [48, 49].

Method- Fluorescein 2% is instilled in the eye. It can be instilled in varying volume and concentrations either by impregnated strips or micropipette. A standardized method is to be followed every time and instructions are given to naturally blink thrice than stop blinking until instructed again [50].

A cut-off of < 10 seconds is used to diagnose DED. In patients of Sjogren syndrome, the sensitivity and specificity of the test have been reported to be 72.2% and 61.6%, respectively [7].

3.3.4.2 Non- invasive tear break-up time (NIBUT)

Tear film stability is believed to be affected by various factors such as temperature, fluorescein dye, humidity, air circulation so NIBUT is more reliable than the other tests.

Method –

- Placido disk -It can be measured with the help of a Placido disk images reflected over the anterior corneal surface with corneal topography systems [51].

- Keratography - Automated assessment is done with instruments having specific software such as keratography which detects and finds the location of tear film break-up over time [52, 53].

- High speed video keratography – The variance of the number of radial rings is estimated form center of the center image [54–56].

- Interferometry – It measures the time between the last blink and the appearance of first discontinuity in the lipid layer of the tear film. Recently instruments measuring the thickness of the lipid layer have also been developed [57–61].
  A cut-off of < 10 seconds is used to diagnose DED. The sensitivity and specificity of the NIBUT is reported to vary according to the technique used, with values of 82–84% and 76–94% respectively [53, 62, 63].

3.3.4.3 Thermography

When the tear film is evaporated it leaves the ocular surface cool [64]. Infrared thermography is used to measure the absolute temperature and the spatial and temporal changes in temperature during the inter-blink period. It can be used as an index of tear film stability.

Purslow and Wolffsohn reported that the ocular surface temperature measured by infrared thermography is related to the tear film [65]. The literature has given many evidences that indicates the cooling rate of the ocular surface is faster in individuals with DED than in normal eyes, which is assumed to be as a result of a greater rate of tear film evaporation [64, 66–68].

3.3.4.4 Osmolarity variability

Osmolarity in the patients of DED varies which in turn affects tear film stability. The inter-eye variability of osmolarity in patients of DED is greater than normal people [69–70]. As the severity of DED increases, this inter-eye difference of osmolarity also increases [71].

3.3.4.5 Tear evaporation rate

It is used as an indicator of tear film stability [72]. Lipid layer is necessary to prevent tear film evaporation. An absent and non-confluent lipid layer of tear film is thought to have association with a 4-fold increase in evaporation rate in normal patients and in patients of keratoconjunctivitis sicca, tear evaporation rate is thought to be increased by 2-fold [73, 74].

Method: Different techniques are used to measure tear film evaporation such as vapor pressure gradient and the velocity of increase in relative humidity (resistance hygrometry) [74–77].

3.3.5 To test the tear evaporation

Goto, Shimazaki et al. in 2002 reported the importance of evaluation of tear evaporation in dry eye assessment [78].

It is a non-invasive procedure and aim at assessing tear dynamics, differentiates the subcategories of DED and evaluating the treatment [79–84]. There are three methods for the measurement:

3.3.5.1 The evaporimeter system

The two humidity sensors are placed at different heights from the ocular surface and they are used to evaluate tear evaporation rates [79].

3.3.5.2 The closed-chamber system

At a given ambient humidity in a closed chamber, the velocity of the humidity increases and it is used to estimate the tear evaporation rate [80–82].

3.3.5.3 The ventilated chamber system

The evaporimeter consists of an eyecup in the form of a ventilated chamber which tightly covers the eye [85].

3.3.6 To test the ocular surface damage

3.3.6.1 Ocular surface staining

Vital and supra-vital stains are used to demonstrate the damaged epithelium. Staining occurs over cornea and conjunctiva in different fashion.

Cornea is stained in manner such that lower part (lower one-third) is stained more than upper part and nasal part stained more than temporal part.

Bulbar conjunctiva is stained nasally and temporally in a wedge-shaped zone [86]. It is a commonly used and cost -effective test.

The dyes used in the procedure are as follows:

- Fluorescein – 1% or 2% commercial preparation is used clinically for the ocular surface staining. It stains the surface when there is a disruption of cell junctions. It stains corneal epithelial damage better than conjunctiva. At physiologic pH, fluorescein is highly water soluble and hence poorly penetrates the lipid layer and doesn't stain normal cornea. It is orange in color and fluoresces green when excited by blue light.
  Yokoi and Kinoshita in 1998 reported that conjunctival damage precedes that of the cornea and is more severe.
  Method – Either it is instilled in form of a drop or impregnated strip. Excess dye is washed off if drop is instilled. Best results are obtained when viewed through a yellow barrier filter (such as Kodak Wratten 12 absorption filter) plus the standard blue exciter filter of the slit lamp [86].
  In the absence of yellow filter, the conjunctival stain is seen poorly.

- Rose Bengal (RB) – It is available as 1% commercial preparation.
  Method – Firstly, topical anesthesia is instilled in the eye to limit stinging with the dye. The dye is then instilled in the lower conjunctival sac. Excess dye is washed off with normal saline.
  The staining is dose-dependent, the more the dose of dye the more is the staining. Rose Bengal stains ocular surface epithelial cells that are unprotected by mucin or glycocalyx, as well as dead or degenerated cells [87].
  However, RB staining has many disadvantages as well which limits its association with dry eye. Schein et al. in 1997 reported that it stains in asymptomatic patients as well and does not correlate with the subjective symptoms [88]. RB causes staining of the Marx's line i.e., the mucocutaneous junctions of the lid margin. And thus, does not seem to have sufficient sensitivity and specificity [89].

- Lissamine Green – It is a synthetic acidic dye that stains similarly to RB. But it is not stringent to the eyes. Staining is dose- dependent. Staining should be checked at a proper time. It should neither be hasty nor be delayed as evaluating the staining too quickly does not allow the staining pattern to develop and if the evaluation is delayed the stain pattern starts fading. Ideally it should be checked between 1 and 4 minutes after staining [90].

- SCORING SYSTEM –

  Most commonly 3 methods are used to grade the ocular surface staining –

- Van Bijsterveld system – This system was developed in 1969. The whole ocular surface is divided into 3 zones – cornea, nasal bulbar conjunctiva and temporal bulbar conjunctiva. Each zone is the scaled from 0 to 3 where 0 indicates no staining and 3 indicates confluent staining. The maximum possible score in 9 [91].

- NEI/Industry Workshop guidelines – This system was developed in 1995. The cornea is divided into 5 sectors namely central, superior, inferior, nasal and temporal, each of them is scored from 0 to 3. The maximum score is 15. Both the nasal and temporal conjunctiva is divided into 3 areas namely superior paralimbal area, inferior paralimbal area and peripheral area, each of which is scored from 0 to 3 with a maximum score of 9 for both nasal and temporal conjunctiva [92].

- Oxford scheme – This scheme was developed by Bron in 2003. There is a chart with series of panels labeled from A-E in order of severity- absent, minimal, mild, moderate and severe [93].

Recently, Miyata and coauthors described a new method for grading fluorescein staining in superficial punctate keratitis (SPK). Both the area and density of SPK were graded. The area was graded from A0 to A3 and the density was graded from D0 to D3 and then these two were combined in a single index [94].

3.3.6.2 Impression cytology

It is used to diagnose diseases like DED, limbal stem-cell deficiency, ocular surface neoplasia, and specific viral infections [95]. In patients of DED, it is used to study squamous metaplasia and goblet cell density of the conjunctiva for the diagnosis and monitoring of the disease [96].

Method - Cells from the first to third most superficial layers of the epithelium are removed by application of cellulose acetate filters or bio-pore membranes, and the cells can be subsequently analyzed by various methods including microscopy, immunocytochemistry, immunoblotting analysis, polymerase chain reaction, and flow cytometry, depending on the aim of the investigation [97].

Several squamous metaplasia grading systems by Nelson, Tseng and Blades are used to analyze the conjunctival impression cytology [98–100].

3.3.6.3 Lid Parallel Conjunctival Folds (LIPCOF)

These are the folds in bulbar conjunctiva in the lateral and lower quadrant which are parallel to the lower lid margin. They represent mild stage of conjuntivochalasis but clinically they are slightly different [101].

The tear meniscus height measurements may be underestimated due to LIPCOF [44].

3.3.6.4 In-vivo confocal microscopy (IVCM)

It is a non-invasive technique to evaluate the signs of ocular surface damage in DED patients at cellular level. The signs such as decreased corneal (apex and lower periphery), and conjunctival epithelial cell density, conjunctival squamous metaplasia (increased mean individual epithelial cell area, decreased nucleocytoplasmic ratio and goblet cell density), and corneal nerve changes (decreased sub-basal nerve density, increased tortuosity and increased number of bead-like formations) are evaluated [102–106].

3.3.6.5 Ocular surface sensitivity

The palpebral conjunctival sensitivity appears to be more critical than corneal sensitivity when assessing DED [107]. The instruments like Cochet-Bonnet or non-contact air-jet esthesiometers have been employed to evaluate ocular surface sensitivity.

3.3.7 To test the lipid layer of the tear film

The precorneal lipid layer assessment is done with the help of tear film interferometry.

The lid margin lipid layer assessment is done with the help of meibometry [108].

The meibomian gland assessment is done with the help of meibography [109].

3.3.7.1 Tear film interferometry

It is a non-invasive method that is used to visualize the translucent surface of the lipid layer of the tear film. McDonald in 1968 was first to analyze the tear interference images [110].

3.3.8 To test the chemical properties of the tear film

3.3.8.1 Tear film osmolarity

Interferon gamma is significantly increased in amount if the tear film on the ocular surface becomes hyperosmolar but other cytokines such as Th1, Th2 and Th17 have no significant increase in amount [111].

It has the highest correlation to disease severity of clinical DED tests [112].

Various literatures have proposed many cut-off values for DED from 305 mOsm/L to 316 mOsm/L [113], with reported sensitivities and specificities ranging from 64–91% and 78–96% respectively [113–117].

3.3.8.2 Tear film ferning

When tear film is dried on a glass plate, it causes ferning. There are few pre requisites for the process such as slow crystal growth rate, low solution viscosity and low impurity levels to permit free-solute diffusion. Seven to ten minutes under normal room temperature of 20 to 26°C and room humidity of (RH up to 50%) has been recommended [118].

The crystallization begins with the formation of a nucleus, due to the supersaturation of ions with solvent evaporation at the peripheral edge of the drop. Normal crystals are formed when the sample solute is able to diffuse into areas with a lower solute concentration [118].

Electrolytes may play a role in ferning as hyperosmolarity has been found to result in deteriorated ferns [113, 119].

Tear ferning changes with contact lens wear have been found to have a moderately high sensitivity (78.4%) and specificity (78.4%) for predicting contact lens tolerance in a clinical setting [120].

Healthy tear samples produce compact, dense ferning patterns, while in dry eye samples, the pattern is fragmented or absent.

3.3.8.3 Biochemical analysis of the tear composition

It includes lacrimal gland and serum protein analysis, mucin analysis and lipid analysis [36].

3.3.9 To test the inflammation of the ocular surface

Inflammation, although not specific, but is a recognized as one of the component of the pathophysiological mechanism of DED.

3.3.9.1 Ocular or conjunctival redness

This is the most common and consistent sign of ocular surface inflammation [121–123]. It can easily be detected with a pen torch or on slit lamp examination. It is not specific to DED and can occur in any disease with inflammation, for example, in response to chemical injury, infective conjunctivitis or allergic conjunctivitis.

3.3.9.2 Matrix metalloproteinases

They are secreted into the tears of a DED patients [72, 124–126]. It destroys the tight junctions of the ocular surface epithelium which in turn leads to loss of ocular surface barrier function. This assay produces a dichotomous outcome, with levels above 40 ng/ml producing a positive result, and is non-specific to the source of ocular surface inflammation.

3.3.9.3 Cytokines and chemokines

They reflect the level of epithelial disease. Elevation of Th1 and Th17 subclasses of cytokines suggest involvement of particular T lymphocyte differentiation pathways in the disease. Elevation of tear Th2 cytokines, on the other hand, may suggest a more allergic-based disease, although recent evidence suggests various aspects of T cell Th1, Th2 and Th17 exist across aqueous deficient, evaporative and mixed forms of DED, with a propensity towards Th1 type T cell responses as a more global indicator of DED [127].

3.3.9.4 Ocular sursface immune markers

The most commonly used ocular surface immune marker is HLA-DR expression, a Class-II MHC antigen, which indicates a loss of the normally immune-suppressed environment of the ocular surface.

Although the authors found increased expression of HLA-DR associated with increased clinical severity of DED [128], but in comparison with other studies the normal levels of HLA-DR expression showed high variability ranging from 5–54% and the study also suggested the weak correlation of HLA-DR and traditional clinical signs of DED [129]. Other relevant markers of apoptosis include CAM-1, CD14+, CD8+ and CD4+ cells [130, 131].

3.3.9.5 In vivo confocal imaging

Corneal sub-epithelial and stromal IVCM signs of inflammation have been hypothesized and studied in DED [132, 133].

4. Clinical protocol for dry eye

The recommended order and clinical practice procedural recommendations are as follows:

- Symptoms - DEQ-5 or OSDI are self-administered. The result is considered positive if the DEQ-5 score is 6 or if OSDI score is 13.

- Tear breakup time

  a. NIBUT - The cut-off for a positive finding can be as low as 2.7 seconds for automated algorithms, and up to 10 seconds for subjective observation techniques.

  b. FBUT - A positive finding has been reported to be a value < 10 seconds.

- Osmolarity - A positive result is considered to be 308 mOsm/L with the currently available device in either eye [69, 71] or an interocular difference >8 mOsm/L [112].

- Ocular surface staining – by lissamine green and fluorescein dye.

Author details

Shrinkhal*, Rupal Verma and Anupam Singh
All India Institute of Medical Sciences, Rishikesh, Uttarakhand, India

*Address all correspondence to: shrinkhalbhu@gmail.com

References

[1] Craig JP, Nichols KK, Nichols JJ, Caffery B, Dua HS, Akpek EK. TFOS DEWS II Definition and Classification Report. Ocul Surf. 2017;**15**:276-283

[2] Schiffman RM, Christianson MD, Jacobsen G, Hirsch JD, Reis BL. Reliability and validity of the ocular surface disease index. Arch Ophthalmol. 2000;118:615-621.

[3] Ozcura F, Aydin S, Helvaci MR. Ocular surface disease index for the diagnosis of dry eye syndrome. Ocular Immunology and Inflammation. 2007;15(5):389-93.

[4] Chalmers RL, Begley CG. The Dry eye questionnaire 5(DEQ-5):Use of a 5-item habitual symptom score to discriminate between groups with varying self-assessed severity. Investigative Ophthalmology and Visual Science. 2008;49(13):5851

[5] Begley CG, Chalmers RL, Abetz L, Venkataraman K, Mertzanis P, Caffery BA. The relationship between habitual patient-reported symptoms and clinical signs among patients with dry eye of varying severity. Invest Ophthalmol Vis Sci. 2003;44:4753-61.

[6] Bjerrum KB. Test and symptoms in keratoconjunctivitis sicca and their correlation. Acta Ophthalmol Scand. 1996;74:436-41.

[7] Vitali C, Moutsopoulos HM, Bombardieri S. The European Community Study Group on diagnostic criteria for Sjogren's Syndrome. Sensitivity and specificity of tests for ocular and oral involvement in Sjogren's syndrome. Ann Rheum Dis. 1994;53:637-47

[8] Begley CG, Caffery B, Chalmers RL, Mitchell GL, Dry Eye Investigation Study G. Use of the dry eye questionnaire to measure symptoms of ocular irritation in patients with aqueous tear deficient dry eye. Cornea. 2002;21:664-70.

[9] Rajagopalan K, Abetz L, Mertzanis P, Espindle D, Begley C, Chalmers R. Comparing the discriminative validity of two generic and one disease-specific health-related quality of life measures in a sample of patients with dry eye. Value Health. 2005;8:168-74.

[10] Li M, Gong L, Chapin WJ, Zhu M. Assessment of vision-related quality of life in dry eye patients. Invest Ophthalmol Vis Sci. 2012;53:5722-7.

[11] Nichols KK, Mitchell GL, Zadnik K. Performance and repeatability of the NEIVFQ-25 in patients with dry eye. Cornea. 2002;21:578-83.

[12] Sakane Y, Yokoi N, Uchino M, Dogru M, Oishi T. Development and validation of the dry eye-related quality-of-life score questionnaire. JAMA Ophthalmol. 2013;131:1331-8.

[13] Gonzalez-Perez M, Susi R, Antona B, Barrio A, Gonzalez E. The ComputerVision Symptom Scale (CVSS17): development and initial validation. Invest Ophthalmol Vis Sci. 2014;55:4504-11.

[14] McMonnies C Ho A Wakefield D. Optimum dry eye classification using questionnaire responses. Adv Exp Med Biol. 1998;438:835-8.

[15] McMonnies CW Ho A. Patient history in screening for dry eye conditions. J Am Optom Assoc. 1987;58:296-301.

[16] Gothwal VK, Pesudovs K, Wright TA, McMonnies CW. McMonnies Questionnnaire: Enhancing screening for dry ete syndromes with Rasch Analysis Investigative Ophthalmology and Visual Science. 2010;51(3):1401-7.

[17] Johnson ME, Murphy PJ. Measurement of ocular surface irritation on a linear interval scale with the ocular comfort index. Investigative Ophthalmology and Visual Science. 2007;48(10):4451-8.

[18] Amparo F, Schaumberg DA, Dana R. Comparison of Two Questionnaires for Dry Eye Symptom Assessment: The Ocular Surface Disease Index and the Symptom Assessment in Dry Eye. Ophthalmology. 2015;122(7):1498-503.

[19] Caffery B, Chalmers RL, Marsden H. Correlation of tear osmolarity and dry eye symptoms in convention attendees. Optom Vis Sci. 2014;91: 142-149.

[20] Begley CG, Caffery B, Nichols KK, Chalmers R. Responses of Contact Lens Wearers to a Dry Eye Survey. *Optometry and Vision Science*. 2000;77(1):40-6.

[21] Nichols JJ, Mithcell GL, Nichols KK, Chalmers R, Begley C. The performance of the contact lens dry eye questionnaire as a screen survey for contact lens-related dry eye. *Cornea*. 2002;21:469-475.

[22] De Boer MR, Moll AC, de Vet HC, et al. Psychometric properties of vision-related quality of life questionnaires: a systematic review. Ophthalmic Physiol Opt. 2004;24:257-273.

[23] Wolffsohn JS, Arita R, Chalmers R, Djalilian A, Dogru M, Dumbleton K, et al. TFOS DEWS II Diagnostic Methodology report. The Ocular Surface. 2017;15:539-74.

[24] Dogru M, Ishida K, Matsumoto Y, Goto E, Ishioka M, Kojima T. Strip meniscometry: a new and simple method of tear meniscus evaluation. Invest Ophthalmol Vis Sci. 2006;47:1895-901.

[25] Ibrahim OM, Dogru M, Ward SK, Matsumoto Y, Wakamatsu TH, Ishida K, et al. The efficacy, sensitivity, and specificity of strip meniscometry in conjunction with tear function tests in the assessment of tear meniscus. Invest Ophthalmol Vis Sci. 2011;52:2194-8

[26] Nelson PS.A shorter Schirmer tear test. Optom Mon. 1982;73:568-9.

[27] Bawazeer AM, Hodge WG. One-minute Schirmer test with anesthesia. 2003.Cornea, 22:285-7.

[28] de Monchy I, Gendron G, Miceli C, Pogorzalek N, Mariette X, Labetoulle M. Combination of the Schirmer I and phenol red thread tests as a rescue strategy for diagnosis of ocular dryness associated with Sjogren's syndrome. Invest Ophthalmol Vis Sci. 2011;52:5167-73.

[29] Cho P. The cotton thread test: a brief review and a clinical study of its reliability on Hong Kong-Chinese. Optom Vis Sci. 1993;70:804-8.

[30] Tomlinson A, Blades KJ, Pearce EI. What does the phenol red thread test actually measure? Optom Vis Sci. 2001;78:142-6.

[31] Miller WL, Doughty MJ, Narayanan S, Leach NE, Tran A, Gaume AL, et al. A comparison of tear volume (by tear meniscus height and phenol red thread test) and tear fluid osmolality measures in non-lens wearers and in contact lens wearers. Eye Contact Lens. 2004;30:132-7.

[32] Sakamoto R, Bennett ES, Henry VA, Paragina S, Narumi T, Izumi Y, et al. The phenol red thread tear test: a cross-cultural study. Invest Ophthalmol Vis Sci. 1993;34:3510-4.

[33] Patel S, Farrell J, Blades KJ, Grierson DJ. The value of a phenol red impregnated thread for differentiating between the aqueous and non-aqueous deficient dry eye. Ophthalmic Physiol Opt-1998;18:471-6.

[34] Pult H, Purslow C, Murphy PJ. The relationship between clinical signs and dry eye symptoms. Eye (Lond). 2011;25:502-10.

[35] Doughty MJ, Whyte J, Li W. The phenol red thread test for lacrimal volumeedoes it matter if the eyes are open or closed? Ophthalmic Physiol Opt. 2007;27:482-9.

[36] Savini G, Prabhawasat P, Kojima T, Grueterich M, Espana E, Goto E. The challenge of dry eye diagnosis. Clinical Ophthalmology. 2008;2(1):31-55.

[37] Jordan A, Baum J. Basic tear flow. Does it exist? Ophthalmology. 1980;87:920-30.

[38] Kaye SB, Sims G, Willoughby C et al. Modification of the tear function index and its use in the diagnosis of Sjögren's syndrome. Br J Ophthalmol. 2001;85:193-9.

[39] Mainstone JC, Bruce AS, Golding TR. Tear meniscus measurement in the diagnosis of dry eye. Curr Eye Res. 1996;15:653-61.

[40] Golding TR, Bruce AS, Mainstone JC. Relationship between tear-meniscus parameters and tear-film breakup. Cornea. 1997;16:649-61.

[41] Chan HH, Zhao Y, Tun TA, Tong L. Repeatability of tear meniscus evaluation using spectral-domain Cirrus(R) HD-OCT and time-domain Visante(R) OCT. Cont Lens Anterior Eye. 2015;38:368-72.

[42] Czajkowski G, Kaluzny BJ, Laudencka A, Malukiewicz G, Kaluzny JJ. Tear meniscus measurement by spectral optical coherence tomography. Optom Vis Sci. 2012;89:336-42.

[43] Ibrahim OM, Dogru M, Takano Y, Satake Y, Wakamatsu TH, Fukagawa K, et al. Application of visante optical coherence tomography tear meniscus height measurement in the diagnosis of dry eye disease. Ophthalmology. 2010;117:1923-9.

[44] Pult H, Riede-Pult BH. Impact of conjunctival folds on central tear meniscus height. Invest Ophthalmol Vis Sci. 2015;56:1459-66

[45] Tittler EH, Bujak MC, Nguyen P, Zhang X, Li Y, Yiu SC, et al. Between-grader repeatability of tear meniscus measurements using Fourier-domain OCT in patients with dry eye. Ophthalmic Surg Lasers Imaging. 2011;42:423-7

[46] Lemp MA, Holly FJ, Iwata S, Dohlman CH. The precorneal tear film. I. Factors in spreading and maintaining a continuous tear film over the corneal surface. Arch Ophthalmol. 1970;83:89-94.

[47] Norn M. Desiccation of the precorneal tear film I. Corneal wetting time. Acta Ophthalmol. 1969;47:865-80.

[48] Mengher LSB, A J, Tonge SR, Gilbert DJ. Effect of fluorescein instillation on the pre-corneal tear film stability. Curr Eye Res. 1985;4:9-12.

[49] Mooi JK, Wang MT, Lim J, Muller A, Craig JP. Minimising instilled volume reduces the impact of fluorescein on clinical measurements of tear film stability. Cont Lens Anterior Eye. 2017.

[50] Johnson ME, Murphy PJ. Measurement of ocular surface irritation on a linear interval scale with the ocular comfort index. Invest Ophthalmol Vis Sci. 2007;48:4451-8.

[51] Liu Z, Pflugfelder SC. Corneal surface regularity and the effect of artificial tears in aqueous tear deficiency. Ophthalmology. 1999;106:939-43.

[52] Best NDL, Wolffsohn JS. Clinical evaluation of the Oculus keratograph. Cont Lens Anterior Eye. 2012;35:171-4.

[53] Hong J, Sun X, Wei A, Cui X, Li Y, Qian T, et al. Assessment of tear film stability in dry eye with a newly developed keratograph. Cornea. 2013;32: 566.

[54] Alonso-Caneiro D, Iskander DR, Collins MJ. Tear film surface quality with soft contact lenses using dynamic-area high-speed videokeratoscopy. Eye Contact Lens. 2009;35:227-31.

[55] Iskander DR, Collins MJ. Applications of high-speed videokeratoscopy. Clin Exp Optom. 2005;88:223-31.

[56] Kopf M, Yi F, Iskander DR, Collins MJ, Shaw AJ, Straker B. Tear film surface quality with soft contact lenses using dynamic videokeratoscopy. J Optom. 2008;1:14-21

[57] Nichols JJ, Nichols KK, Puent B, Saracino M, Mitchell GL. Evaluation of tear film interference patterns and measures of tear break-up time. Optom Vis Sci. 2002;79:363-9.

[58] Doane MG. An instrument for in vivo tear film interferometry. Optom Vis Sci. 1989;66:383-8.

[59] Guillon JP. Use of the Tearscope Plus and attachments in the routine examination of the marginal dry eye contact lens patient. Adv Exp Med Biol. 1998;438:859-67.

[60] Maissa C, Guillon M. Tear film dynamics and lipid layer characteris-ticseeffect of age and gender. Cont Lens Anterior Eye. 2010;33:176-82.

[61] Yokoi N, Komuro A. Non-invasive methods of assessing the tear film. Exp Eye Res. 2004;78:399-407.

[62] Mengher LS, Bron AJ, Tonge SR, Gilbert DJ. A non-invasive instrument for clinical assessment of the pre-corneal tear film stability. Curr Eye Res. 1985;4:1-7.

[63] Downie LE. Automated tear film surface quality breakup time as a novel clinical marker for tear hyperosmolarity in dry eye disease. Invest Ophthalmol Vis Sci. 2015;56:7260-8.

[64] Craig JP, Singh I, Tomlinson A, Morgan PB. The role of tear physiology in ocular surface temperature. Eye (Lond). 2000;14(Pt 4):635-41.

[65] Purslow C, Wolffsohn J. The relation between physical properties of the anterior eye and ocular surface temperature. Optom Vis Sci. 2007;84: 197-201.

[66] Fujishima H, Toda I, Yamada M, Sato N, Tsubota K. Corneal temperature in patients with dry eye evaluated by infrared radiation thermometry. Br J Ophthalmol. 1996;80:29-32.

[67] Kamao T, Yamaguchi M, Kawasaki S, Mizoue S, Shiraishi A, Ohashi Y. Screening for dry eye with newly developed ocular surface thermographer. Am J Ophthalmol. 2011;151:782-91.

[68] Su TY, Hwa CK, Liu PH, Wu MH, Chang DO, Su PF. Noncontact detection of dry eye using a custom designed infrared thermal image system. J Biomed Opt. 2011;16

[69] Jacobi C, Jacobi A, Kruse FE, Cursiefen C. Tear film osmolarity measurements in dry eye disease using electrical impedance technology. Cornea. 2011;30: 1289-92.

[70] Gilbard JP, Farris RL, Santamaria II J. Osmolarity of tear microvolumes in keratoconjunctivitis sicca. Arch Ophthalmol. 1978;96:677-81.

[71] Lemp MA, Bron AJ, Baudouin C, Benitez Del Castillo JM, Geffen D, Tauber J, et al. Tear osmolarity in the diagnosis and management of dry eye disease. Am J Ophthalmol. 2011;151. 792-8.

[72] Willcox MDP, Argüeso P, Georgiev GA, Holopainen JM, Laurie GW, Millar TJ, et al. TFOS DEWS II Tear Film Report. Ocul Surf. 2017;15:366-403.

[73] Craig JP, Tomlinson A. Importance of the lipid layer in human tear film stability and evaporation. Optom Vis Sci. 1997;74:8-13.

[74] Rolando M, Refojo MF, Kenyon KR. Increased tear evaporation in eyes with keratoconjunctivitis sicca. Arch Ophthalmol. 1983;101:557-8.

[75] Rolando M, Refojo MF. Tear evaporimeter for measuring water evaporation rate from the tear film under controlled conditions in humans. Exp Eye Res. 1983;36:25-33.

[76] Tsubota K, Yamada M. Tear evaporation from the ocular surface. Invest Ophthalmol Vis Sci. 1992;33:2942-50.

[77] Tomlinson A, Cedarstaff TH. Tear evaporation from the human eye: the effects of contact lens wear. J Br Contact Lens Assoc. 1982;5:1416-7.

[78] Goto E, Shimazaki J, Monden Y. Low-concentration homogenized castor oil eye drops for noninfl amed obstructive meibomian gland dysfunction. Ophthalmology. 2002;109:2030-5.

[79] Hamano H, Hori M, Mitsunaga S. Application of an evaporimeter to the fi eld of ophthalmology. J Jpn Contact Lens Soc. 1980;22:101-7

[80] Rolando M, Refojo MF. Tear evaporimeter for measuring water evaporation rate from the tear fi lm under controlled conditions in humans. Exp Eye Res. 1983;36:25-33.

[81] Tsubota K, Yamada M. Tear evaporation from the ocular surface. Invest Ophthalmol Vis Sci. 1992;33:2942-50.

[82] Mathers WD. Ocular evaporation in meibomian gland dysfunction and dry eye. Ophthalmology. 1993;100:347-51.

[83] Shimazaki J. Definition and criteria of dry eye. Ganka. 1995;37:765-70.

[84] Shimazaki J, Goto E, Ono M. Meibomian gland dysfunction in patients with Sjogren syndrome. Ophthalmology. 1998;105:1485-8

[85] Goto E, Endo K, Suzuki A. Tear evaporation dynamics in normal subjects and subjects with obstructive meibomian gland dysfunction. Invest Ophthalmol Vis Sci. 2003;44:533-9

[86] Bron AJ. Diagnosis of Dry Eye. Survey of Ophthalmology. 2001;45(2).

[87] Norn MS: Dead, degenerate, and living cells in conjunctival fluid and mucous thread. Acta Ophthalmol (Copenh). 1969;47: 1102-15.

[88] Schein OD, Tielsch JM, Munoz B. Relation between signs and symptoms of dry eye in the elderly: a population-based perspective. Ophthalmology. 1997;104:1395-1401.

[89] Norn MS. Vital staining of the canaliculus lacrimalis and the palpebral border (Marx' line). Acta Ophthalmol (Copenh). 1966;44:948-59

[90] Foulks GN. Challenges and pitfalls in clinical trials of treatments for dry eye. Ocul Surf. 2003;1:20-30.

[91] Van Bijsterveld OP. Diagnostic tests in the sicca syndrome. Arch Ophthalmol. 1969;82:10-4.

[92] Lemp MA. Report of the National Eye Institute/Industry Workshop on clinical trials in dry eye. CLAO J. 1995;21:221-32.

[93] Bron AJ, Evans VE, Smith JA. Grading of corneal and conjunctival staining in the context of other dry eye tests. Cornea. 2003;22:640-50.

[94] Miyata K, Amano S, Sawa M. A novel grading method for superficial punctate keratopathy magnitude and its correlation with corneal epithelial permeability. Arch Ophthalmol. 2003;121:1537-9.

[95] Tole DM, McKelvie PA, Daniell M. Reliability of impression cytology for the diagnosis of ocular surface squamous neoplasia employing the Biopore membrane. Br J Ophthalmol. 2001;85:154-8.

[96] Mrugacz M, Kasacka I, Bakunowicz-Lazarczyk A, Kaczmarski M, Kulak W. Impression cytology of the conjunctival epithelial cells in patients with cystic fibrosis. Eye (Lond). 2008;22:1137-40.

[97] Brignole F, Pisella PJ, De Saint Jean M, Goldschild M, Goguel A, Baudouin C. Flow cytometric analysis of inflammatory markers in KCS: 6-month treatment with topical cyclopsporin A. Invest Ophthalmol Vis Sci. 2001;42:90-5

[98] Nelson JD, Havener VR, Cameron JD. Cellulose acetate impressions of the ocular surface. Dry eye states. Arch Ophthalmol. 1983;101:1869-72.

[99] Tseng SC. Staging of conjunctival squamous metaplasia by impression cytology. Ophthalmology. 1985;92: 728-33.

[100] Blades K, Doughty MJ, Patel S. Pilot study on the use of impression cytology specimens for quantitative assessment of the surface area of bulbar conjunctival cells. Optom Vis Sci. 1998;75:591-9.

[101] Pult H, Tosatti SGP, Spencer ND, Asfour J-M, Ebenhoch M, Murphy PJ. Spontaneous blinking from a tribological viewpoint. Ocul Surf. 2015;13: 236-49.

[102] Erdelyi B, Kraak R, Zhivov A, Guthoff R, Nemeth J. In vivo confocal laser scanning microscopy of the cornea in dry eye. Graefes Arch Clin Exp Ophthalmol. 2007;245:39-44.

[103] Villani E, Magnani F, Viola F, Santaniello A, Scorza R, Nucci P, et al. In vivo confocal evaluation of the ocular surface morpho-functional unit in dry eye. Optom Vis Sci. 2013;90:576-86.

[104] Wakamatsu TH, Sato EA, Matsumoto Y, Ibrahim OM, Dogru M, Kaido M, et al. Conjunctival in vivo confocal scanning laser microscopy in patients with Sjogren syndrome. Invest Ophthalmol Vis Sci. 2010;51:144-50.

[105] Villani E, Galimberti D, Viola F, Mapelli C, Ratiglia R. The cornea in Sjogren's syndrome: an in vivo confocal study. Invest Ophthalmol Vis Sci. 2007;48: 2017-22.

[106] Kojima T, Matsumoto Y, Dogru M, Tsubota K. The application of in vivo laser scanning confocal microscopy as a tool of conjunctival in vivo cytology in the diagnosis of dry eye ocular surface disease. Mol Vis. 2010;16:2457-64.

[107] Cox SM, Nichols JJ. Association between meibomian gland testing and ocular surface sensitivity. Cornea. 2015;34:1187-92

[108] Chew CKS, Jansweijer C, Tiffany JM. An instrument for quantifying meibomian lipid on the lid margin: the Meibometer. Curr Eye Res. 1993;12:247-54.

[109] Robin JB, Jester JV, Nobe J. In vivo transillumination biomicroscopy and photography of meibomian gland dysfunction. Ophthalmology. 1985;92: 1423-6.

[110] McDonald JE. Surface phenomena of tear films. Trans Am Ophthalmol Soc. 1968;66:905-39.

[111] Jackson DC, Zeng W, Wong CY, Mifsud EJ, Williamson NA, Ang CS, et al.

Tear interferon-gamma as a biomarker for evaporative dry eye disease. Invest Ophthalmol Vis Sci. 2016;57:4824-30

[112] Sullivan BD, Whitmer D, Nichols KK, Tomlinson A, Foulks GN, Geerling G, Khanal S, Ramaesh K, Diaper C, McFadyen A. Tear film osmolarity: determination of a referent for dry eye diagnosis. Invest Ophthalmol Vis Sci. 2010;47:4309-15

[113] Versura P, Profazio V, Campos EC. Performance of tear osmolarity compared to previous diagnostic tests for dry eye diseases. Curr Eye Res. 2010;35:553-64

[114] Versura P, Profazio V, Campos EC. Performance of tear osmolarity compared to previous diagnostic tests for dry eye diseases. Curr Eye Res. 2010;35: 553-64

[115] Schargus M, Ivanova S, Kakkassery V, Dick HB, Joachim S. Correlation of tear film osmolarity and 2 different MMP-9 tests with common dry eye tests in a cohort of non-dry eye patients. Cornea. 2015;34:739-44.

[116] Schargus M, Meyer-ter-Vehn T, Menrath J, Grigoleit GU, Geerling G. Correlation between tear film osmolarity and the disease score of the international chronic ocular graft-versus-host-disease consensus group in hematopoietic stem cell transplantation patients. Cornea. 2015;34:911-6.

[117] Khanal S, Tomlinson A, McFadyen A, CDiaper. Dry eye diagnosis. Invest Ophthalmol Vis Sci. 2008;49:1407-14.

[118] Masmali AM, Purslow C, Murphy PJ. The tear ferning test: a simple clinical technique to evaluate the ocular tear film. Clin Exp Optom. 2014;97: 399-406.

[119] Masmali AM, Al-Qhtani S, Al-Gasham TM, El-Hiti GA, Purslow C, Murphy PJ. Application of a new grading scale for tear ferning in non-dry eye and dry eye subjects. Cont Lens Anterior Eye. 2015;38:39-43.

[120] Ravazzoni L, Ghini C, Macri A, Rolando M. Forecasting of hydrophilic contact lens tolerance by means of tear ferning test. Graefes Arch Clin Exp Ophthalmol. 1998;236:354-8

[121] Papas EB. Key factors in the subjective and objective assessment of conjunctival erythema. Invest Ophthalmol Vis Sci. 2000;41:687-91.

[122] Fieguth P, Simpson T. Automated measurement of bulbar redness. Invest Ophthalmol Vis Sci. 2002;43:340-7.

[123] Amparo F, Wang H, Emami-Naeini P, Karimian P, Dana R. The Ocular Redness Index: a novel automated method for measuring ocular injection. Invest Ophthalmol Vis Sci. 2013;54:4821-6.

[124] Acera A, Rocha G, Vecino E, Lema I, Duran JA. Inflammatory markers in the tears of patients with ocular surface disease. Ophthalmic Res. 2008;40:315-21.

[125] Chotikavanich S, de Paiva CS, Li de Q, Chen JJ, Bian F, Farley WJ, et al. Production and activity of matrix metalloproteinase-9 on the ocular surface increase in dysfunctional tear syndrome. Invest Ophthalmol Vis Sci. 2009;50:3203-9.

[126] Hadassah J, Bhuvaneshwari N, Rao U, Sehgal PK. Evaluation of succinylated collagen bandage lenses in corneal healing by the expression of matrix metalloproteinases (MMP-2 and MMP-9) in tear fluid. Ophthalmic Res. 2009;42:64-72

[127] Meadows JF, Dionne K, Nichols KK. Differential profiling of t-cell cytokines as measured by protein microarray across dry eye subgroups. Cornea. 2016;35: 329-35.

[128]] Epstein SP, Gadaria-Rathod N, Wei Y, Maguire MG, Asbell PA. HLA-DR expression as a biomarker of inflammation for multicenter clinical trials of ocular surface disease. Exp Eye Res. 2013;111:95-104.

[129] Baudouin C, Liang H, Riancho L, Ismail D, Deniaud M, Amrane M, et al. Correlation between the inflammatory marker HLA DR and signs and symptoms in moderate to severe dry eye disease. Invest Ophthalmol Vis Sci. 2015;56. 298.

[130] Sanchez MA, Arriola-Villalobos P, Torralbo-Jimenez P, Giron N, de la Heras B, Herrero Vanrell R, et al. The effect of preservative-free HP-Guar on dry eye after phacoemulsification: a flow cytometric study. Eye (Lond). 2010;24:1331-7.

[131] Guyette N, Williams L, Tran MT, Than T, Bradley J, Kehinde L, et al. Comparison of low-abundance biomarker levels in capillary-collected nonstimulated tears and washout tears of aqueous-deficient and normal patients. Invest Ophthalmol Vis Sci. 2013;54:3729-37.

[132] Mantopoulos D, Cruzat A, Hamrah P. In vivo imaging of corneal inflammation: new tools for clinical practice and research. Semin Ophthalmol. 2010;25:178-85.

[133] Mastropasqua L, Nubile M, Lanzini M, Carpineto P, Ciancaglini M, Pannellini T, et al. Epithelial dendritic cell distribution in normal and inflamed human cornea: in vivo confocal microscopy study. Am J Ophthalmol. 2006;142:736-44.

Section 2

Dry Eye Syndrome: Relationships with Other Ocular Diseases and Treatments

Chapter 5

Glaucoma and Dry Eye

Mauricio Aguirre Baez and Rodrigo Castillo Iturria

Abstract

Glaucoma treatment is closely related to the appearance or worsening of dry eye symptoms. The current topical treatment produces chronic inflammation that affects globet cells, meibomian glands and cornea, which translates into a decrease in the quantity and quality of the tear. It is characterized by increased osmolarity, which perpetuates damage to the ocular surface. Preservatives currently play a fundamental role in damage the ocular surface. There are numerous studies that have shown their toxic effects on the eye. Currently there are numerous preservative-free formulations and new therapies that allow us to improve the condition of the ocular surface in patients with glaucoma. A rational treatment is proposed using the different approaches available in the literature.

Keywords: Dry eye, Glaucoma, tear film, benzalkonium chloride

1. Introduction

Glaucoma is known to be a major cause of optic neuropathy that eventually leads to loss of vision. This is characterized by loss of retinal ganglion cells and their axons, excavated appearance of optic nerve head, and progressive loss of visual field sensitivities.

Quigley and colleagues published pooled-data analyses of glaucoma prevalence. In 2020, 80 millions of people are affected by glaucomatous optic neuropathy [1], of these, 60% will present concomitant ocular surface disease.

There is considerable evidence to suggest that medical treatment of glaucoma contributes to ocular surface disease (OSD) and the development of dry eye [2]; its prevalence with or without symptoms ranges from 5–50%, and the prevalence based on symptoms alone is very higher around 75% [3].

The cause of OSD in glaucoma patients is believed to be multifactorial and may include both the active component of the drug and the preservative, most commonly benzalkonium chloride (BAK), which is capable of causing inflammation and other anterior segment eye diseases that they range from allergy, blepharitis, dry eye, and anatomical eyelid abnormalities [3–5].

2. Mechanisms of damage

2.1 Inflammatory changes with topical treatment

The damage that occurs with topical treatment in glaucoma is the result of chronic inflammatory changes. A significant increase in macrophages, mast cells and lymphocytes has been found in conjunctival biopsies, compared with biopsies of patients who have not received treatment. A significant increase in inflammatory markers has also been found, specifically IgE and Class II HLA-DR1 antigen. All of this suggests that topical treatment produces an inflammatory state on the ocular surface and even on the tenon. This was published in 1989 by Dr. Sherwood, he showed than this inflammatory state affects both the conjunctiva and the tenon [6]. Fibroblasts also were more prominent in the deeper conjunctiva and Tenon's capsule, this finding might be expected to enhance the risk of external bleb scarring after trabeculectomy or valve surgery. Also, this study, in patients who received long-term antiglaucomatous medical therapy, detected a significant decrease in the number of goblet cells in patients who received long-term antiglaucomatous medical therapy, this contributes to dry eye in glaucoma patients, in addition to other studies have explored the potential association between topical anti-glaucoma medications and meibomian gland dysfunction [7].

2.2 Meibomian gland dysfunction in Glaucoma

We know that Meibomian gland dysfunction (MGD) is a chronic diffuse eyelid margin disease that is associated with tear film instability, inflammation, and OSD. MGD is the most common cause of evaporative dry eye. The mechanism underlying the changes in the meibomian glands is unclear, some studies have reported that results by a chronic inflammation of the conjunctiva, altered by long-term anti-glaucoma eye drop use [6]. These chronic inflammation causes morphological and functional changes in the glands. Some studies have shown stagnation of meibum followed by the keratinization of orifices in the meibomian glands [8]. Arita et al., using non-contact meibography, compares a Two treated group with control, subgroup analysis revealed than the meibomian gland loss in the PG-treated eyes and β-blocker-treated eyes, that was significantly higher than in the corresponding controls [9].

2.3 Changes in extracellular matrix

In extracellular matrix (ECM) a pair of enzyme families called the matrix metalloproteinases (MMPs; a group of enzymes catalyzing the degradation of ECM) and the tissue inhibitors of metalloproteinase (TIMPs) are involved in the regulation and maintenance of the ECM. MMPs and TIMPs are involved in physiological mechanisms. ECM accumulation caused by changes of MMP and TIMP expression is significantly involved in the increased outflow resistance in glaucomatous eyes and changes in ECM metabolism of ocular surface tissue, specifically changes in conjunctival tissues, including a decrease in the number of epithelial goblet cells, and increase in subepithelial collagen deposition [10].

The topical treatment for glaucoma can cause damage to the ocular surface where different inflammatory pathways, which over time affect the globet cells and Meibomian glands among other ocular structures. This damage is due to both, the components of the drugs and the preservatives, of which the most used is BAK, However many studies indicate a direct correlation between the presence of preservatives and the symptoms experienced during antiglaucoma therapy. Most effects observed in glaucoma patients are therefore more likely to be due to the preservative than the active ingredients [11], however, It has been described specific alterations in the ocular surface from each family of drugs.

3. Clinical manifestation of specific medications on ocular surface

3.1 Prostaglandin analogs

Are the most powerful and efficient agents for controlling intraocular pressure among all current ocular hypotensive medications [12]. Latanoprost has been shown to induce squamous metaplasia, to stimulate HLA-DR overexpression at the conjunctival surface, and to cause significant changes in the metalloproteinase and tissue inhibitor balance [10, 13].

Conjunctival hyperemia is the earliest and most notorious side effect. The hyperemia is due to vasodilatation and not from an allergic reaction, as seen with other drug classes. This manifestation is more marked during the first month of use.

3.2 Beta-blockers

The Beta-blockers, for many physicians, is the second choice for controlling intraocular pressure, has been shown ocular discomfort due to burning, hyperemia, toxic keratopathy, superficial punctate keratopathy (SPK), periocular contact dermatitis, and dry eye [14].

SPK was the most common finding with surface staining. It was reported in 6% of patients using timolol.

Other reported effects of timolol is the decreases tear production. This effect is quantitatively limited and does not appear dangerous for normal eyes, although it may become so for eyes with an originally low lacrimal secretion [15].

3.3 α Adrenergic Agonists

Ocular surface the effects include ocular allergy, conjunctival follicles. Allergic reaction has been observed in up to 15% in chronic treatment with brimonidine [14].

3.4 Carbonic anhydrase inhibitors

Ocular surface side effects include allergic conjunctivitis and periorbital dermatitis [14].

4. The role of Benzalkonium chloride (BAK)

Benzalkonium chloride (BAK) has been used in ophthalmology since the 1940s. It is by far most common preservative, found in approximately 70% of eye drops while only 10% use other preservatives. It is used in different concentrations varied from 0.005% to 0.02% [16]. It is a quaternary ammonium compound that acts as a detergent, lysing cell membranes and thus killing microorganisms [17], in this way prevents bacterial and fungal contamination in multidose eye drop containers. It is highly effective as a preservative. It was also initially thought that the detergent effect of BAK might be necessary for the penetration of the active ingredient.

BAK toxicity for eye structures has been reported in many studies, in experimental or cell models have consistently and reliably shown its toxic effects. One major argument that is proposed to maintain the use of quaternary ammoniums in eyedrop formulations is that BAK reportedly enhances the penetration of the drug into the anterior chamber, through disruption of the hydrophobic barrier of the corneal epitheliumm [18], however there are a large number of non-inferiority studies for bak free drugs that demonstrate the effectiveness of these medications.

4.1 Bak toxicity in globet cells

Low doses of BAK can induced proapoptotic efect on conjutival cells lines involving, as shown in vitro, reactive oxygen species and, therefore, oxidative stress reducing the number of goblet cells [19]. This cytotoxicity was proportional to the BAK concentration. In an interesting study by Guenoun, it was shown that these effects can be neutralized by topical prostaglandins analogs [20].

4.2 Corneal toxicity

Like the conjunctiva, the corneal cells have shown similar apoptotic response to BAK in superficial and deeper layers. Liang et al. confirmed the cytotoxicity of BAK in a model of a 3D culture of corneal epithelium. This study confirmed that BAK, depending on the time and concentration used, acts as a pro-inflammatory and pro-apoptotic agent able to impair the normal epithelium turnover irreversibly, even after BAK withdrawal [21].

Other study has been show topical application of BAK to the eye causes neurotoxicity, this secondarily produces reduction in aqueous tear production. Cessation of BAK treatment leads to resolution of inflammation, normalization of tear production, and recovery of stromal nerve density [22].

The damage to the ocular surface (conjuntiva, globet cells, Meibomian gland dysfunction and cornea) by topical treatment manifests itself with dry eye symptoms that have been described more frequently with the use of BAK. Jaenen et al. show a very high Prevalence of symptoms in patients using preserved drops, with 43% discomfort upon instillation, 40% burning or stinging sensation, 31% foreign body sensation, 23% dry eyes, 21% tearing, and 18% itchy eyelids [11]. Clinical impairment of the tear film and a rapid decrease of goblet cell density were also demonstrated after starting treatment with preserved timolol [22]. Schirmer's test and break-up time were altered compared to the basal control already significantly in the first month of treatment ($P < 0.01$ and $P < 0.001$, respectively). Similarly, impression cytology showed a progressive decrease in goblet cell density also significant at the first month.

5. Tear production and surface staining

The alteration of glaucoma medications affect the globet cells and meibomian glands affecting the tear film, both in quantity and quality [23]. This is accompanied by increased osmolarity.

Hyperosmolarity stimulates a cascade of inflammatory events in the epithelial surface cells, involving MAP kinases and NFkB signaling pathways and the generation of inflammatory cytokines (IL-1A; -1B; TNF-A) and MMPs (MMP9), which arise from or activate inflammatory cells at the ocular surface, these inflammatory events lead to apoptotic death of surface epithelial cells, including goblet cells, as already explained. In this way, a vicious circle is created that began with the topical treatment and is perpetuated over time. Clearly there are other factors such as the existence of previous ocular surface disease and individual variability that can give a wide range of symptoms [24].

6. Management of ocular surface disease in patient with Glaucoma: general perspective

Currently there are numerous bak-free drugs, laser therapy and minimally Invasive Glaucoma Surgery (MIGS) that help us in the management of the ocular surface and also improve adherence to therapy. The adherence and persistence is a problem, between 30 to 70% of patients do not comply with the indications in the management of glaucoma [25], in large part it is due to the irritative symptoms that these eyedrops produce.

Gupta et al. in his study shows that 90% of patients do not instillate the Eye drop properly [26]. The new advances in glaucoma therapy are focused on improving adherence and persistence with the aim of preserving the ocular surface and slowing the progression of the disease.

The bak-free medicine maintains an antimicrobial environment in a multidose container while minimizing toxicity to the ocular surface. The major disadvantage of preservative-free therapy is its cost and the handling of these containers, is often difficult for patients squeze the bottle, many of them have double chambers that avoid microbial contamination.

Selective laser trabeculoplasty (SLT) reduces intraocular pressure by increasing aqueous outflow through the trabecular meshwork with a single, painless outpatient laser procedure, minimal recovery time, and good safety profile. The Light study found that 74% of patients randomized to initial SLT remained drop-free at 36 months, suggesting that SLT is a particularly effective treatment in treatment-naïve patients [27].

MIGS have been developed as safer and less traumatic surgical interventions for patients with mild to moderate glaucoma or who are intolerant to standard medical therapy. It is an excellent option to avoid the use of topical medications. The problem of the MIGS continues to be accessibility; the high costs make them often prohibitive as a therapeutic option in developing countries.

Intense pulsed light therapy (IPL) is a promising complementary treatment for dry eye disease, specifically when dry eye syndrome is associated with skin disorders. Recent studies demonstrated in patients suffering from meibomian gland dysfunction (MGD), IPL therapy also reduces signs and symptoms of ocular surface disease [28]. The biological basis of this process is not well understood. The mechanism of action is by photomodulation that induces intracellular changes at the ducts of meibomian glands. There are no conclusive studies of its exact utility in patients with dry eye and glaucoma, however it may be a tool to consider [29].

6.1 Management of ocular surface disease in patient with Glaucoma

The classic management of glaucoma must be relationated with the Ocular surface evaluation. It's known the low % of glaucoma eye drops adherence. Recognize and make objective evaluations of the ocular surface can provide vital information about our patients. It can help to stratify the initial baseline therapy, and propose a double objective. Achieve the target IOP and the best Ocular surface condition in all patients.

There are two complementary forms of evaluate the ocular surface condition; Subjective, using validated questionnaires. These test evaluate the symptoms and how the patients confront the environment with the disease. Objective methods, is a standardized test to evaluate the cornea and conjunctival epithelium, and the tear film osmolarity.

- Subjective evaluation

  Validated questionaries

- Objective evaluation

  a. Ocular vital tinctions

  b. Osmolarity

  - Tearlab
  - Ipen

  c. Inflamation marker

  d. No contact measurements

  - Lacrydiag
  - Keratograph

6.2 Subjective evaluation: questionnaires

6.2.1 Ocular surface disease index (OSDI)

The OSDI test evaluates the symptoms provided by the patient and the function affection related to vision [30]. This 12-item questionnaire assesses dry eye symptoms and the effects it has on vision-related function in the past week of the patient's life [31]. The questionnaire has 3 subscales: ocular symptoms, vision-related function, and environmental triggers. Different Scores are provided related to the severity of ocular surface disease [32].

6.2.2 Standard patient evaluation of eye dryness questionnaire (SPEED)

The SPEED questionnaire was designed to make a rapid evaluation of dry eye symptoms [33]. It assesses whether these symptoms were not problematic, tolerable, uncomfortable, bothersome, or intolerable [34]. Also monitored diurnal and symptoms changes over 3 months [35]. The sensitivity and specificity of SPEED test versus OSDI were 0.90 and 0.80 respectively [35].

6.2.3 DEQ 5

The DEQ-5 consists of five questions that assess discomfort and dryness intensity. The overall DEQ-5 was calculated by summing the score on the individual questions. The reliability of the overall OSDI and DEQ-5 scores were 0.919 and 0.819 respectively [36].

6.3 Objetive measurements

6.3.1 Schirmer test (ST)

The Shirmer Test 1 (ST-1) is performed without instilling proparacaine i.e. topical anesthetic (reflex tear secretion), ST-2 after instilling proparacaine (basic tear secretion).

6.3.2 Non invasive tear break up time

The stained cornea is examined under the slit lamp in cobalt blue filter, the observer evaluate the appearance of first dry spot on cornea in less than 10 seconds. If this event occurs, its indicative of evaporative dry eye [37].

6.3.3 Ocular surface punctate staining

The observar stained cornea with fluorescein sodium and conjunctiva with lissamine green. Appearance of >5 corneal spots or > 9 conjuntival spot and lid margin (2 mm length & 25% width) seen under cobalt blue light is indicative of dry eye [37].

6.4 Osmolarity

6.4.1 Tear lab osmometer

Osmolarity testing has been declared the "gold standard" of objective dry eye diagnosis. Cutoff value >308 mOsm is indicative of hiperosmolarity state, and compatible with dry eye.

6.4.2 IPEN

The cut off value of 318 mOsm/L showed a sensitivity of 90.9% and specificity of 90.6% for diagnosing DED. The IPen osmometer can be considered suitable for use in the clinical setting, with good performance in DED diagnosis [38].

6.5 Inflamation test

INFLAMMADRY: Inflamma Dry is a rapid, in-office test that detects elevated levels of MMP-9, an inflammatory marker which is consistently elevated in the tears of patients with DED [39].

6.6 No contact evaluation

There are new devices at our disposal, which can evaluate and perform an adequate evaluation of the ocular surface. We explain two of them (No commercial interest). With these reports, the physician can explain an show the different characteristics altered in the test. This unique feature can improve the adherence to treatment.

- **Lacrydiag (Quantel)** [40] Reports available.
    - NIBUT (No invasive brake up time).
    - Lacrimal meniscus height.
    - LIPID LAYER INTERFEROMETRY - Measures lipid layer thickness and accurately diagnoses and monitors lipid-deficient tear.
    - MEIBOGRAPHY: Specialized imaging study developed exclusively for the purpose of directly visualizing the morphology of meibomian gland, they play a significant role in tear production by contributing lipids to the superficial tear film and hence dysfunction of the meibomian glands results EDE.

- **Keratograph** (Oculus) [41] Reports available.
    - o NIBUT.
    - o Lacrimal meniscus height.
    - o LIPID LAYER INTERFEROMETRY - Measures lipid layer thickness and accurately diagnoses and monitors lipid-deficient.
    - o MEIBOGRAPHY: Specialized imaging study developed exclusively for the purpose of directly visualizing the morphology of meibomian gland, they play a significant role in tear production by contributing lipids to the superficial tear film and hence dysfunction of the meibomian glands results EDE.

Management proposal

Once the glaucoma is diagnosed or we evaluate our patients in control, and recognize subjective or objective symptoms or signs, an escalated treatment is proposed. Our goal is **provide an adequate treatment, looking for no glaucoma progression with the minimal or none ocular discomfort.**

7. Treatment

Before initiating treatment, a careful evaluation of the ocular surface and periocular structures is mandatory. Its importan observe if any other alterations of the periocular structures are compromised, in example: lid malposition, rosacea, blepharitis, allergies, among the important. These alterations must me treated aiming to relieve the ocular surface [42]. In presence of early signs or symptoms of OSD are recognized (scores and/or objective evaluations), treatment must be initiated.

7.1 Evaluation of glaucoma treatment

As a general principle, the physician must evaluate, if it is possible, to:

1. Suspend Bak preservatives eyedrops
2. Promote use combined presentations
3. Evaluate use of SLT as initial treatment or MIGS.

7.2 Ocular surface management: basic treatment

7.2.1 Non preserved eyedrops

Cochrane reviews reports no difference in OTC (over the counter) artificial tears [43]. Preserved agents use alternative preservatives to BAK and may be considered because of the decreased cost, increased availability, and the convenience of standard multi-dose containers, non-preserved agents are preferred and should be considered wherever possible [44].

7.2.2 Heating devices

External eyelid heating devices have demonstrated efficacy in reducing surface staining scoring, improving TBUT and meibomian gland secretions, optimally with continued 2 times per day applications of $\geq$5 minútese [45, 46].

7.2.3 Eyelid hygiene

Its recommended by the authors, it must be evaluated the presence of Demodex or signs of rosacea. There are diverse options for treatment. Some products containing tree tea oil [52].

7.2.4 Omega 3 fatty acid supplementation

Omega-3 fatty acid supplementation significantly improved OSD symptoms and signs [47].

7.2.5 Lipidic substitutes eyedrops

Is used when a lipid deficiency is detectected, (Rosacea), meibomian gland disfunction. They are developed to enhance the lipidic layer of the tear-film, by different substances. Comercial eyedrops available are Systaine Balance and Optive Advance (no commercial interest) [48].

7.3 Ocular surface advance treatment

Ciclosporine % (Restasis) [49]:
Cochrane: studies support the topical CsA may increase the number of conjunctival goblet cells- FDA Approved

- Indication: Dry eye moderate
- Dosage: BID

Lifetigrast 5% (Xidra) [50]:

- Indication Dry eye FDA Approved
- Dosage: BID

Serum tears: [51].

- Indication: Second line, dry eye management.
  Different concentrations, usually 20%.
  Cochrane revision: no sufficient information.
- Dosage: QUID

7.4 Ocular surface estabilization

Other authors recommend suspend the topical glaucoma treatment and use topical steroids to evaluate the reincorporation of treatment and provide oral acetazolamide for the IOP control.

7.5 Local antinflamatory measures

7.5.1 Tea oil tree eyelid

- Indication: eyelid irritation Demodex follicullorum, demodex brevis
- Dosage: nocturnal use [52].

7.5.2 External eyelid brush

- Indication: Moderate Dry eye. Blepharitis, rosácea, Meibomian gland dysfunction.

- Dosage: 1 time/week [53].

7.5.3 Infrared pulse light (IPL)

- Indication: Moderate Dry eye. Blepharitis, rosácea, Meibomian gland dysfunction.

- Dosage: Different schedules provided by the manufacturer [29].

7.6 Surgery

It must be indicated as the first therapy, which depends of the conjunctival damage and glaucoma severity. This point is still on debate in the actual literature.

8. Author's recommendation

- Consider initiating preservative free topical medications or surgical/procedural alternatives such as laser trabeculoplasty, minimally invasive glaucoma surgery, or novel forms of drug delivery in all cases where possible and even more, if there is a previous ocular surface disease present.

- In all patients with maximum tolerated medical therapy, it is ideal to indicate eyelid cleanliness.

- Maximizing the health of the ocular surface may be another treatment option that is viable for some patients. Utilizing artificial tears with sodium hyaluronate or hydroxypropyl-methycellulose/dextran, both ocular surface lubricants, can provide some relief of ocular surface disease symptoms.

- In patients with an allergy reaction to different families of topical medications, it must be considered that there may be an allergic reaction to BAK.

- The reduction of irritative symptoms when switching to therapy without bak, generally occurs after three months of use.

- Topical cyclosporine 0.05% twice daily in conjunction with glaucoma drops if another preventative and ocular surface modifying measure, specifically if the patient had a filtering surgery.

Author details

Mauricio Aguirre Baez* and Rodrigo Castillo Iturria
Department of Ophthalmology, Hospital Barros Luco-Trudeau, Santiago, Chile

*Address all correspondence to: pacinodoc@gmail.com

References

[1] Quigley HA, Broman AT. The number of people with glaucoma world-wide in 2010 and 2020. Br J Ophthalmol. 2006;90:262-7.

[2] Anwar Z, Wellik SR, Galor A. Glaucoma therapy and ocular sur-face disease: current literature and recommendations. Curr Opin Ophthalmol 2013;24:136Y43.

[3] Stewart WC, Stewart JA, Nelson LA. Ocular surface disease in patients with ocular hypertension and glaucoma. Curr Eye Res 2011;36:391e8.

[4] Baudouin C, Labbé A, Liang H, et al. Preservatives in eye-drops: The good, the bad and the ugly. Prog Retin Eye Res. 2010;29:312-334.

[5] Fechtner RD, Godfrey DG, Budenz D, Stewart JA, Stewart WC, Jasek MC. Prevalence of ocular surface complaints in patients with glaucoma using topical intraocular pressure-lowering medications. Cornea 2010;29:618Y21.

[6] Sherwood MB, Grierson I, Millar L, Hitchings RA. Long-term morphologic effects of antiglaucoma drugs on the conjunctiva and tenon's capsule in glaucomatous patients. Ophthalmology. 1989; 96(3):327-335. [PubMed: 2710524]

[7] Uzunosmanoglu E, Mocan MC, Kocabeyoglu S, Karakaya J, Irkec M. Meibomian gland dysfunction in patients receiving long-term glaucoma medications. Cornea 2016;35:1112e6.

[8] Nicolaides N, Santos EC, Smith RE, Jester JV (1989) Meibomian gland dysfunction, III: meibomian gland lipids. Invest Ophthalmol Vis Sci 30:946-951.

[9] Arita, R., Itoh, K., Maeda, S., Maeda, K., Furuta, A., Tomidokoro, A., Amano, S. (2012). Effects of long-term topical anti-glaucoma medications on meibomian glands. Graefe's Archive for Clinical and Experimental Ophthalmo logy, 250(8), 1181-1185.

[10] Ito T, Ohguro H, Mamiya K, et al. Effects of antiglaucoma drops on MMP and TIMP balance in conjunctival and subconjunctival tissue. Invest Ophthalmol Vis Sci 2006;47:823-30.

[11] Jaenen, N., Baudouin, C., Pouliquen, P., Manni, G., Figueiredo, A., Zeyen, T., 2007. Ocular symptoms and signs with preserved and preservative-free glaucoma medications. Eur. J. Ophthalmol. 17, 341-349

[12] Parrish RK, Palmberg P, Sheu WP, XLT Study Group. A comparison of latanoprost, bimatoprost, and travoprost in pa-tients with elevated intraocular pressure: a 12-week, random-ized, masked-evaluator multicenter study. Am J Ophthalmol 2003;135:688-703.

[13] Baudouin, C., Liang, H., Hamard, P., Riancho, L., Creuzot-Garcher, C., Warnet, J.-M., & Brignole-Baudouin, F. (2008). The Ocular Surface of Glaucoma Patients Treated over the Long

[14] JoAnn, A. & Law, S.K. & Coleman, A.L. & Nouri-Mahdavi, Kouros & Caprioli, Joseph. (2016). Pearls of Glaucoma Management: Second Edition.

[15] Bonomi L, Zavarise G, Noya E, Michieletto S. Effects of timolol maleate on tear flow in human eyes. Albrecht Von Graefes Arch Klin Exp Ophthalmol. 1980;213(1):19-22. doi: 10.1007/BF02391207. PMID: 6906142.

[16] Rasmussen CA, Kaufman PL, Kiland JA. Benzalkonium chloride and glaucoma. J Ocul Pharmacol Ther 2014;30:163-9.

[17] Tripathi, B.J., Tripathi, R.C., and Killi, S.P. Cytotoxicity of ophthalmic preservatives on human corneal epithelium. Lens Eye Toxic Res. 9:361-337, 1992.

[18] Baudouin, C., Riancho, L., Warnet, J.M., Brignole, F., 2007. In vitro studies of anti-glaucomatous prostaglandin analogues: travoprost with and without benzal-konium chloride and preserved latanoprost. Invest. Ophthalmol. Vis. Sci. 48, 4123e4128.

[19] Faria NVL, Sampaio MOB, Viapiana GN, Seabra NM, Russ HH, Montiani-Ferreira F, Mello PAA. Effects of benzalkonium chloride and cyclosporine applied topically to rabbit conjunctiva: a histomorphometric study. Arq Bras Oftalmol. 2019 Jul-Aug;82(4): 310-316.

[20] Guenoun JM, Baudouin C, Rat P, et al. In vitro comparison of cytoprotective and antioxidative effects of latanoprost, travoprost, and bimatoprost on conjunctiva-derived epithelial cells. Invest Ophthalmol Vis Sci 2005;46: 4594-9.

[21] Liang H, Pauly A, Riancho L, et al. Toxicological evaluation of preservative-containing and preservative-free topical prostaglandin analogues on a three-dimensional-reconstituted corneal epithelium system. Br J Ophthalmol 2011;95:869-75.

[22] Joy Sarkar, Shweta Chaudhary, Abed Namavari, Okan Ozturk, Jin-Hong Chang, Lisette Yco, Snehal Sonawane, Vishakha Khanolkar, Joelle Hallak, Sandeep Jain; Corneal Neurotoxicity Due to Topical Benzalkonium Chloride. Invest. Ophthalmol. Vis. Sci. 2012;53(4):1792-1802.

[23] Herreras, J.M., Pastor, J.C., Calonge, M., Asensio, V.M., 1992. Ocular surface alteration after long-term treatment with an antiglaucomatous drug. Ophthalmology 99, 1082e1088.

[24] The definition and classification of dry eye disease: report of the Definition and Classification Subcommittee of the International Dry Eye WorkShop (2007). Ocul Surf. 2007 Apr;5(2):75-92.

[25] Friedman DS, Quigley HA, Gelb L, Tan J, Margolis J, Shah SN, Kim EE, Zimmerman T, Hahn SR. Using pharmacy claims data to study adherence to glaucoma medications: methodology and findings of the Glaucoma Adherence and Persistency Study (GAPS). Invest Ophthalmol Vis Sci. 2007 Nov;48(11):5052-7.

[26] Gupta R, Patil B, Shah BM, Bali SJ, Mishra SK, Dada T. Evaluating eye drop instillation technique in glaucoma patients. J Glaucoma. 2012 Mar;21(3):189-92.

[27] Gazzard G, Konstantakopoulou E, Garway-Heath D, et al. Selective laser trabeculoplasty versus eye drops for first-line treatment of ocular hypertension and glaucoma (LiGHT): a multicentre randomised controlled trial. Lancet. 2019;393: 1505e1516.

[28] Dell SJ. Intense pulsed light for evaporative dry eye disease. *Clin Ophthalmol*. 2017;11:1167-1173. Published 2017 Jun 20. doi:10.2147/OPTH.S139894

[29] Cote S, Zhang AC, Ahmadzai V, Maleken A, Li C, Oppedisano J, Nair K, Busija L, Downie LE. Intense pulsed light (IPL) therapy for the treatment of meibomian gland dysfunction. Cochrane Database Syst Rev. 2020 Mar 18;3(3):CD013559.

[30] Schiffman RM. Reliability and Validity of the Ocular Surface Disease Index. *Archives of Ophthalmology.* 2000;*118*(5):615-621.

[31] Bottomley A, Jones D, Claassens L. Patient-reported outcomes: Assessment and current perspectives of the guidelines of the Food and Drug

Administration and the reflection paper of the European Medicines Agency. *European Journal of Cancer.* 2009;*45*(3): 347-353.

[32] Grubbs JR, Tolleson-Rinehart S, Huynh K, Davis RM. A Review of Quality of Life Measures in Dry Eye Questionnaires. *Cornea.* 2014;*33*(2): 215-218.

[33] Blackie C, Albou-Ganem C, Korb D. Questionnaire assists in dry eye disease diagnosis. Four-question survey helps evaluate patients' dry eye symptoms to improve screening. *Ocular Surgery News* Europe Edition. 2012.

[34] Asiedu K. Rasch Analysis of the Standard Patient Evaluation of Eye Dryness Questionnaire. *Eye & Contact Lens: Science & Clinical Practice.* 2017;43(6):394-398.

[35] Ngo W, Situ P, Keir N, Korb D, Blackie C, Simpson T. Psychometric properties and validation of the Standard Patient Evaluation of Eye Dryness questionnaire. *Cornea.* 2013;*32*(9):1204-1210.

[36] Chalmers RL, Begley CG, Caffery B. Validation of the 5-Item Dry Eye Questionnaire (DEQ-5): discrimination across self-assessed severity and aqueous tear deficient dry eye diagnoses. Contact Lens Anterior Eye 2010;33:55-60.

[37] Wolffsohn JS, Arita R, Chalmers R, et al. TFOS DEWS II Diagnostic Methodology report. Ocul Surf. 2017;15(3):539-574.

[38] Park, J., Choi, Y., Han, G. *et al.* Evaluation of tear osmolarity measured by I-Pen osmolarity system in patients with dry eye. *Sci Rep* **11,** 7726 (2021). https://doi.org/10.1038/s41598-021-87336-2

[39] Sambursky R. Presence or absence of ocular surface inflammation directs clinical and therapeutic management of dry eye. Clin Ophthalmol. 2016 Nov 24;10:2337-2343. doi: 10.2147/OPTH.S121256. PMID: 27920494; PMCID: PMC5127432

[40] J Fr Ophtalmol 2021 Mar;44(3):313-320. doi: 10.1016/j.jfo.2020.06.045. Epub 2021 Feb 11.

[41] Evaluation of tear film and meibomian gland function in dry eyepatients using Keratograph 5M. Zhejiang Da Xue Xue Bao Yi Xue Ban2016 May 25;45(4):422-428.

[42] Jones L, Downie LE, Korb D, et al. TFOS DEWS II management and therapy report. Ocul Surf. 2017; 15:575-628.

[43] https://doi.org/10.1002/14651858.CD009729.pub2

[44] Grene RB, Lankston P, Mordaunt J, et al. Unpreserved carboxymethylcellulose artificial tears evaluated in patients with keratoconjunctivitis sicca. Cornea. 1992;11:294-301.

[45] Arita R, Morishige N, Shirakawa R, et al. Effects of eyelid warming devices on tear film parameters in normal subjects and patients with meibomian gland dysfunction. Ocul Surf. 2015;13: 321-330.

[46] Blackie CA, Solomon JD, Greiner JV, et al. Inner eyelid surface temperature as a function of warm compress methodology. Optom Vis Sci. 2008;85:675-683.

[47] Giannaccare G, Pellegrini M, Sebastiani S, et al. Efficacy of omega-3 fatty acid supplementation for treatment of dry eye disease: a meta-analysis of randomized clinical trials. Cornea. 2019;38:565-573.

[48] Moshirfar M, Pierson K, Hanamaikai K, Santiago-Caban L,

Muthappan V, Passi SF. Artificial tears potpourri: a literature review. Clin Ophthalmol. 2014 Jul 31;8:1419-33. doi: 10.2147/OPTH.S65263.

[49] de Paiva CS, Pflugfelder SC, Ng SM, Akpek EK. Topical cyclosporine A therapy for dry eye syndrome. Cochrane Database of Systematic Reviews 2019, Issue 9. Art. No.: CD010051. DOI: 10.1002/14651858.CD010051.pub2

[50] Pflugfelder SC, de Paiva CS. The Pathophysiology of Dry Eye Disease: What We Know and Future Directions for Research. Ophthalmology. 2017 Nov;124(11S):S4-S13. doi: 10.1016/j.ophtha.2017.07.010. PMID: 29055361; PMCID: PMC5657523.

[51] Pan Q, Angelina A, Marrone M, Stark WJ, Akpek EK. Autologous serum eye drops for dry eye. Cochrane Database of Systematic Reviews 2017, Issue 2. Art. No.: CD009327. DOI: 10.1002/14651858.CD009327.pub3.

[52] Savla K, Le JT, Pucker AD. Tea tree oil for Demodex blepharitis. Cochrane Database of Systematic Reviews 2020, Issue 6. Art. No.: CD013333. DOI: 10.1002/14651858.CD013333.pub2.

[53] Xie, W. J., Jiang, L. J., Zhang, X., Xu, Y. S., & Yao, Y. F. (2019). Eyelid margin cleaning using Deep Cleaning Device for the treatment of meibomian gland dysfunction-associated dry eye: a preliminary investigation. *Journal of Zhejiang University. Science. B*, *20*(8), 679-686. https://doi.org/10.1631/jzus.B1900091

Chapter 6

How Ocular Surface Disorder Affected Corneal Graft Survival

Sharita Siregar

Abstract

The ocular surface is formed by three component tissues: The cornea, conjunctiva, and limbus all play an important role in keeping a good and clear corneal graft. As part of non-immunological reactions, glaucoma and ocular surface disorders can increase the possibility of corneal graft failure. For that reason, maintaining a healthy and moist ocular surface, depends on an intimate relationship between healthy ocular surface epithelia, the tear film, and the eyelid, which will all increase corneal graft survival. A moist conjunctiva composed of lymphatic tissue as our defense mechanism against infection, will keep the cornea avascular, remaining crystal clear, dehydrated, and protected. Ocular surface epithelium cannot survive without tears. To specified, each component tissue that forms the ocular surface is equally important. Several previous studies revealed that dry eye disease as a form of ocular surface disorders (OSD), can lead to graft rejection. To our knowledge, there are two conditions that cause dry eye syndrome. It can be caused by lipid tear deficiency or aqueous tear deficiency. The severity of dry eye also ranges widely with some mild inflammatory processes leading to severe chronic conditions (i.e., cicatrizing conjunctivitis) that are known to be an absolute contraindication for total or full penetrating keratoplasty. The basic immunological mechanism of dry eye, as one of the most forms of ocular surface disorders that altered corneal graft survival will be discussed specifically in this chapter.

Keywords: Ocular surface disorder, dry eye disease, corneal graft survival, immune privilege, immunopathology, dendritic cells, inflammation, cornea

1. Introduction

Cornea transplantation is considered the most successful form of organ allo-transplantation. Immune privilege has been found to be responsible for the high rate of cornea graft survival. Cornea avascularity as well the absence of lymph nodes suppresses antigen transportation and presentation to naive T cells. The spectrum of neuropeptides and complement activation from the cornea combined with aqueous humor immune tolerance - also known as anterior chamber associated immune deviation (ACAID) - will make the cornea tissue become more adaptable and not easily responsive to any foreign antigen from the graft tissue [1, 2]. However, any form of inflammation, vascularization, infection, or previous graft failure will be considered high risk factors that cause rejection due to an adaptive immune response [3]. Loss of graft survival can be defined as a condition where the cornea loses its transparency after two weeks of clarity and is considered a failure if cornea edema persists at six months. Moreover, if in six months persistent graft edema remains unclear after treatment with a high dose immunosuppressive agent, it should be considered an irreversible rejection. On the other hand, it will be considered a reversible rejection if the graft reaches its clarity after successful treatment [4].

Cornea infection is considered a high-risk factor for corneal transplant rejection. No matter what causes the infection, any form of bacterial, fungal, and viral infection is recognized as factors that increase the risk for graft rejection. Several conditions like a poor ocular surface, coexisting allergies, trauma, or previous intraocular surgeries can disrupt and make conditions worse and accelerate the likely risk of developing graft failure [5–7].

Dry eye disease (DED) that affects tens of millions of people worldwide, is one of the most common types of ocular surface disorders which may initiate graft failure through an immunopathological response [8, 9]. Tear hyperosmolarity is also found to play a major role in the vicious cycle of dry eye disease that is associated with activation of inflammation [10]. Japanese researchers assessed that a DED cornea donor tissue acts as a significant risk factor for subsequent corneal allograft rejection. They found that donor corneas from patients with DED will activate inflammation by augmenting T-cells at the host, promoting dendritic cell maturation in the cornea and draining lymph nodes of the host, increased Th1 and Th17 frequencies and decreased Treg function in the recipient and this activates host T cells through a direct pathway of allosensitization. Therefore, the possibility of a cornea transplant recipient who received donor material from a patient with moderate to severe dry eye disease may predispose higher rejection rates in the grafted host [11].

Recipient characteristics such as the recipient's indication for grafting, previous glaucoma drainage implant surgery and which type of keratoplasty technique performed may profoundly affect the number of endothelial cells lost and graft survival as well. Although there is depth of tissue differences in the amount of implanted cornea tissue between endothelial keratoplasty (EK) and posterior keratoplasty (PK), the endothelial cell loss was found to be similar [12] during 10 years of follow up (71% for EK vs. 78% for PK).

2. Incidence

To estimate the possibility of corneal transplants being rejected, a good explanation about what is allograft rejection and when we can define a condition as a cornea graft failure are needed. The term cornea graft rejection refers to a specific immune response from the recipient after the donor tissue was transplanted and characterized by a successful clear cornea graft condition for two weeks following cornea transplantation. Graft failure is defined as primary graft failure if cornea edema was found to exist immediately after it was transplanted, and it never reached clarity. Any improper cornea tissue storage or surgical trauma can cause graft failure. The immune system is found to give a huge role in the graft tissue to develop rejection or failure. A previous study concluded that cornea transplant success not only depends on the donor and recipient tissue condition, but it also depends on what type of keratoplasty, and which immune pathway is involved (direct or indirect) [13].

The status of donor cornea conditions that are correlated with graft survival rates was studied in 2018. It was reported that donor tissue with a history of dry eye disease will cause a higher number in APCs from the recipient ocular surface draining lymph nodes (dLNs), induce the maturation of dendritic cells and show an increase in the number of CD4 effector T cells produced that will reduce the graft survival rate to 10% [11, 14].

In the same study, at two weeks after surgery, it was also found that an increase in interferon-γ (IFN-γ) and cytokine interleukin 17 (IL_17) secretion and a reduced number Foxp3 expression will interfere with the T regulatory cells ability to protect graft tissue from the recipient's immune response and can lead to rejection [15–18]. In conclusion, cornea graft survival rate is an estimated rate during a period of time that the graft tissue is able to maintain its clarity after transplantation. The successful and high cornea graft survival rate is related not only to its immune privilege but also the status of the recipient bed such as the amount of cornea tissue replaced (penetrating or lamellar keratoplasty), the underlying disease, the amount of vascularization, the presence of glaucoma, inflammation, the number of regrafts performed and larger graft size.

The study done by Eghtedari reported that during a 5-year period, DALK gave better graft survival rates compared to DSAEK and PK in terms of corneal regrafting with a percentage of 1.2% compared to 5% and 8.25%. It is believed because the endothelial layer was not included for the DALK procedure. The primary disease of the cornea that led to transplantation is also proposed to be an important factor in future graft survival and important indicators such as infection (bacterial, herpetic, and fungal) being the major cause of graft rejection and need for repeat grafting (35%), with pseudo phakic bullous keratopathy as the second most common factor with 30.3% chances for corneal regraft. Other risk factors that determine graft survival are as follows: First, the quality of the donor cornea itself where a lower quality donor cornea that was used for tectonic purposes showed a lower survival rate compared to a higher quality donor cornea in keratoplasty for optical reasons. Secondly, glaucoma was found to be responsible for about 13% of regrafts cases. As for corneal vascularization, the existence of pannus was found in 25% of regrafts which is similar to the 10-year previous study that showed the graft survival rates of 35 to 40%. The immune privilege that normally is present in the cornea was interfered with by the lower impression of T regulatory cells caused by a small number of Foxp3 factors expressed [3, 18].

3. The vicious circle of dry eye

Tear hyperosmolarity is the core mechanism of dry eye disease (DED). The cause of DED can be divided into two forms, aqueous-deficient dry eye (ADDE) and evaporative dry eye (EDE). In ADDE, tear hyperosmolarity results when lacrimal secretion is reduced, with the normal process of evaporation from the eye. In EDE, tear hyperosmolarity is caused by excessive evaporation from the exposed tear film in the presence of a normally functioning lacrimal gland. Since tear osmolarity can only rise because of tear evaporation in both ADDE and EDE, tear hyperosmolarity is due to evaporation from the ocular surface and in that sense, all forms of DED are evaporative. EDE is a hyper-evaporative state. In DED, tear hyperosmolarity is considered to set up a cascade of signaling events within surface epithelial cells, that leads to the release of inflammatory mediators and proteases. Any etiology that induces an increase in tear hyperosmolarity will eventually create an ocular surface disorder. This in turn can activate each inflammatory mediator as a compensatory response.

As a disease caused by multiple factors, dry eye disease is characterized by the loss of homeostasis in the tear film along with ocular symptoms. Intercellular adhesion molecule (ICAM-1) is an over expressed and attracted lymphocyte function associated antigen-1 (LFA-1) receptor that is located at the surface of T cells can either be activated or inactivated. If ICAM-1 binds to LFA-1 receptor, it will release cytokine and cause the inactivated T cell to become activated. The higher amount of cytokine release, the higher number of activated T cells which leads to more severe tissue inflammation occurs [19, 20].

4. Immunopathological mechanisms

There are two kinds of immune systems, the first is also known as an innate immune system consisting of a component that is already in the location and responds immediately after it is exposed, with a general response. As for specific immune system response, it is formed by T cells and B cells that are located far from the exact location of the stimulus and launched with a specialized system after it is triggered after multiple stimuli.

4.1 Overview of immune responses in dry eye

4.1.1 Innate immune responses

As mentioned previously, the innate immune response is a fast and nonspecific immune response that is created by the ocular surface as a protection from any microbial invasion or toxin passage across its surface epithelium. Facilitated by the mucin layer of the tears, the glycocalyx changes at the conjunctiva, together with the cornea epithelium, along with production of a stream of antimicrobial defense proteins such as lysozyme, lipocalin, lactoferrin and trefoil peptides, makes the corneal and conjunctival epithelium considered as the "gatekeepers" of the ocular surface [21–25].

The hyperosmolar state of the tear film will also activate MAPK kinases and its master regulator NFkB. This regulator will produce interleukin-1 (IL-1) and TNF-α that will up-regulate matrix metalloproteinase-9 (MMP-9) and associated with disruption of the epithelial cornea barrier [26]. The activation of pattern recognition receptors (PRRs) such as the Toll-like receptors (TLRs) and the NOD-like receptors (NLR) will create an inflammatory response towards DED as part of innate immune response [27]. Induction in chemokines by the ocular surface will attract macrophages, dendritic cells, neutrophils and activated T cells [28–33]. Moreover, blood vessel endothelial cells will produce an adhesion molecule called intracellular adhesion molecule-1 (ICAM-1) in DED [34]. This ICAM-1 will bind to inflammatory cells and express an integrin leukocyte function antigen-1 (LFA-1) causing migration and activation at the site of inflammation and lymphoid organs [35].

4.1.2 Adaptive immune responses

Accumulation of CD11c antigen presenting cells maturation and the activation of antigen specific CD4+ T cells in draining lymph nodes during desiccating stress, with the reduction of CD4+ T cell infiltration numbers in depleted macrophages was found as evidence that can explain why the ocular surface antigen presentation was considered as the first initiator of adaptive immune response [36]. The upregulation in major histocompatibility complex II (MHC II) and primed T cells that are recruited to a patient's cornea and conjunctiva in DED found were also considered as another plausible pathway in local adaptive immune responses [37, 38]. Keep in mind that adaptive immune systems are evolving and becoming more specific through time by memorizing the first encounter antigen.

4.2 Corneal immune responses

4.2.1 Immune privilege of the cornea

Because cornea is avascular and lymphatic free, the graft survival rate for corneal transplantation is the highest among all other organ transplants and this condition is often referred to as immune privilege of the cornea. Dendritic cells which are also known as the messenger cells of the immune system in cornea graft tissue, exist in an immature inactivated state which will result in immune quiescence in a healthy cornea. All cornea layers are found to have a very low expression of MHC class I and II antigens, limiting immunogenicity to foreign antigens. The transport of antigens and APCs to T cell-rich secondary lymphoid organs as a part of the immune system do not happen in the cornea because of its absence of lymph vessels. Cell membrane bound molecules are also expressed by the cornea - for instance Fas Ligand (FasL), MHC-Ib, tumor necrosis factor (TNF) and complement regulatory protein (CRP). These molecules guard from immune mediated inflammation and induce apoptosis of immune effector cells. FasL expressed by corneal epithelium and endothelium acts as a pro apoptotic molecule. It also will destroy polymorphonuclear neutrophils (PMNs) and effector T cells that express its receptor Fas/CD95, creating immune quiescence while protecting the cornea from immune mediated graft rejection [39, 40]. The corneal epithelium and stroma produce programmed death ligand-1 (PD-L1) which interacts with its receptor PD-1 on the T cells and leads to inhibition of T cells proliferating, induction of apoptosis and suppression of interferon (IFN-γ) secretion [41], promoting graft survival [42, 43].

Soluble immunosuppressive factors inside the anterior chamber will inhibit T cell and complement activation [44, 45]. This alloantigen specific peripheral immune tolerance from aqueous humor is also known as anterior chamber associated immune deviation (ACAID) which modulate the systemic cytotoxic immune response [46, 47] and suppresses delayed-type hypersensitivity. Therefore, ACAID also known as a factor that promote graft survival [48, 49].

4.2.2 Immunopathology of corneal graft rejection

All cells of each living individual express a surface polymorphic protein antigen also known as major histocompatibility complex (MHC) antigens that are located at chromosome 6. The variations in MHC genes are the reason why everyone has their own characteristic hence differentiate people one to another. Therefore, if the antigen between the donor and the recipient was mismatched, the recipient will directly reject the allograft tissue.

Human leukocyte antigen (HLA) is responsible for MHC expression [50]. There are two types of class for MHC expression. MHC type I (MHC-1) is found on all nucleated cells of the body and platelets. In the cornea, its antigens are expressed by corneal epithelial, stromal, and endothelial cells. These transmembrane glycoproteins are coded for HLA-A, -B and -C genes. As for MHC type II (MHC-II) is more specific compared to class I. It was limited only at the cell surface of immunocompetent antigen-presenting cells (APCs) like DCs, macrophages and Langerhans cells [51].

Foreign antigens carried by APCs and presented to naive T cells with the presence of MHC-II will stimulate molecules and recognize it as a non-self-antigen. Any inflammation, interferon gamma and surgery will induce the expression of MHC II antigens even more in the cornea [52].

Dendritic cells as the messenger of the immune system will bring the foreign antigen from their exact location of inflammation and transport them to the lymph node which will activate B cells at the spleen and T cells at the thymus glands. It is known that corneal DCs play a critical role in graft rejection through their ability to regulate T cell response to both self and foreign antigens of the cornea donor tissue.

Antigen was recognized by the MHC class II at the surface of mature DCs. After it binds to its receptor at the surface of T cell/CD4, they will cause the replication of T cells into several types of T cells. The first type is T helper. Antigen that was present to it will be recognized by the CD8 and cause cytokine release. After cytokine release, T helper will differentiate into a cytotoxic T cell.

The second type of T cell is found actively in plasma cells differentiation into antibodies and create an immune memory at the first encounter antigen. It will recall a similar response every time the same pathogen exists. The third type is the T cell that will release cytokine to attract monocytes and macrophages at the inflammation site so the phagocytosis process can occur.

The role of dendritic cells in graft rejection was determined by regulating the T cells after the antigen was presented and recognized by the MHC class II antigen receptor at the surface of mature DC. Normally, these central corneal DCs will remain silent, dormant, and undifferentiated. However, any kind of stress like inflammation will activate DCs and after the DC reaches the cornea through bloodstream where the donor alloantigen was captured by lymphoid organs, it will be transported and presented back into T cell for further immune response [53].

5. Dry eye disease predilection to corneal graft rejection

Patients with dry eye disease will complain about foreign body sensation, blurred vision, and redness on their eyes due to the lack of tear production and rapid tear evaporation caused by poor tear stability as their characteristic. The lacrimal gland dysfunction creates an inflamed ocular surface, and it is considered as the pathognomonic sign of DED [54].

Post corneal graft patients often will develop ocular dryness as a side effect from consuming glaucoma medication that can lead to poorer healing process at the ocular surface. The mechanisms of the poorer healing process are as follows. Dryness at the ocular surface activates inflammatory mediators such as collagenase and will create a defect at the epithelium of the cornea if it was not treated which can lead to an infection or induce vascularization that can affect as a high-risk factor for corneal graft rejection [55]. Tear examination may show shorter tear break-up time (BUT) and an unstable tear film.

Glaucoma is the adverse effect because of long-term steroid topical medication usage. Contrarily, steroid eye drops are also very important to prevent graft rejection in post corneal transplant patients. Each glaucoma medication has their own mechanism in causing any cornea or ocular surface disorder. For example, beta blocker eye drops like timolol has been found to act on the beta receptors on lacrimal gland that will reduce basal tear turnover rate after one month of therapy [56]. Prostaglandin analog medication will obstruct the meibomian gland even more [57]. Brimonidine tartrate as the alpha-adrenergic agonist mostly used may predispose the patient into ocular allergy [58]. Although corneal thickness has been found to be related to carbonic anhydrase inhibitor brinzolamide eye drop, further investigation is still needed [59]. Ocular surface disease because of the long-term glaucoma medication use is related to the increment of macrophages found in the conjunctiva. The expression of inflammatory marker like antigen HLA-DR and Immunoglobulin E is higher in patient with prolonged glaucoma topical medication compared to untreated eyes [60–62].

LASIK as one of refractive surgery procedures will cause ocular dryness through the laser dissection at the corneal nerves that will interrupt the corneal reflex arc further and reduce the tear film production with substance P release which will increase the severity of inflammation [63, 64].

The mechanism in DED related post refractive surgery was thought to be similar to DED followed by perforating keratoplasty. The whole dissected corneal nerve using trephination in keratoplasty will release substance P because all corneal nerves are dissected during trephination. Substance P from keratocytes [65] will induce the secretion of interleukin 8 as a pro inflammatory chemokine. Kuchle et al. demonstrated that dry eye disease is a risk factor for graft rejection in PK through inflammatory mechanisms [66].

6. Treatment of corneal graft rejection

6.1 Provide a healthy ocular surface

A smooth ocular surface can be achieved through intensive and frequent non-preserved tear supplements or hyaluronate eye drops [67]. Frequent drops using non-preserved tears is necessary for managing accumulated inflammatory cytokines. Hyaluronate eye drops have been reported to be effective in managing patients with ocular surface disorders through improving the corneal epithelial barrier function, promoting corneal wound healing, and reducing ocular surface tissue damage as well as minimizing the inflammation process in DED [68].

Epithelial rejection occurred at the first three months after surgery can be seen as a linear opacification at the cornea surface which stains with fluorescein. Although the dead epithelial cells are replaced rapidly by recipient epithelial cells, it is important to remember that these recipient epithelial cells have been sensitized by the donor which can progress to deeper rejection such as stromal or endothelial rejection in the future. It can be seen as a nummular infiltrate if the rejection reaches the stroma. However, endothelial rejection can be shown as keratic precipitates where the inflammatory cells adhere to the endothelial graft [69].

6.2 Immunosuppressive agents

Topical steroid eye drops such as dexamethasone 0.1% or prednisolone acetate 1% are given every three hours per day for the first 2–3 months, then tapered gradually until it reaches zero in one year. These steroid drop regimens are different for each center. The purpose of steroid drops is to prevent and reverse any rejection episodes and avoid more endothelial cell loss. Lack of detecting signs of rejection will postpone graft treatment initiation. Delay in diagnosing or treating rejection will reduce graft sensitivity towards the treatment and may develop to an irreversible rejection [70, 71].

6.3 HLA matching

HLA matching is shown to be effective in predicting graft survival rates in a vascularized organ allotransplantation. However, the benefits from tissue matching in cornea transplantation are still debatable since the cornea has its own immune privilege as a non-vascularized tissue. Nevertheless, it was found that an active graft rejection is related to the donor HLA class I specific cytotoxic T cells.

The greater number of mismatches between HLA-A and HLA-B shows a higher risk of corneal tissue developing into graft rejection. These tissue mismatches are considered as a high-risk factor for rejection after corneal transplantation [72–76]. Whilst Collaborative Corneal Transplantation Studies (CCTS) suggest the necessity of HLA matching in corneal transplantation remains doubtful, it may be useful for high-risk patients although it is still not considered to do the tissue matching as part of routine preoperative assessment due to the donor cornea tissue available [77].

Minor histocompatibility antigens such as ABO blood antigens are a different class of cell surface proteins that are also expressed by the corneal epithelium. It is coded throughout the genome at various loci [78]. CCTS concluded with ABO blood matching, the possibility for someone having graft rejection is 41% if the ABO antigens are incompatible and 31% may experience rejection for the compatible ABO antigens. The study concluded ABO matching may still be considered useful in predicting corneal graft rejection. However, doing HLA matching is still debatable - not only because of the lack in the availability of cornea tissue globally but also its very expensive [79].

7. Conclusion and future prospects

Cornea graft survival rates are influenced by many factors. Dry eye as part of ocular surface disorders is one important thing that we should care for. The aim for dry eye or OSD management is to treat the hyperosmolarity condition of the tear film to reduce the expression of a response from our immune system to any foreign antigens from desiccating stress or inflammation. Although the cornea has immune privilege due to being avascular and lymph node free, a successful prevention of immune rejection is better compared to immune suppression by immune modifying treatments such as gene therapy post transplantation. Minor histocompatibility complex tissue matching can be done due to its low cost. However, ABO antigens testing is not as specific as major histocompatibility tests.

Cornea as the only organ that has its own immune privilege is still in doubt for testing major histocompatibility complex tissue matching. Mainly, because most of major histocompatibility testing only work for class II but not shown effective for class I. Unfortunately, due to human major histocompatibility complex genes are highly polymorphic, any random allocation of HLA will achieve the required matching level in a very long time which are very unethical for our patients. If in the future, there will be a HLA matching that is highly specific, low cost and only needs a period of time to get the test result, probably the HLA testing can be applied as a routine evaluation to provide higher number of graft survival in the future.

As mentioned in the literature, a high-risk condition such as corneal vascularization, DED and prolonged use of antiglaucoma medication can reduce the corneal graft survival rate. Therefore, the application of anti VEGF through injection on the subconjunctival, an adjunct non-preservative topical lubricant in glaucoma medication and the use of lifitegrast as the antagonist of LFA-1 and inhibits T cell formation in dry eye management will probably useful and create a promising result related to a higher graft survival rate in the future.

To conclude, a prospective clinical trial to investigate the role of preexisting DED in the context of corneal transplantation and its influence on graft survival is needed. Understanding the role of HLA in corneal graft rejection from an immunological point of view as well as the necessity of conducting a comprehensive knowledge of the HLA tissue matching will create other options to prevent graft rejection. Future pharmacotherapies for DED with novel targets are the focus of ongoing research, and several promising treatment options are expected.

Acknowledgements

The author would like to thank Professor John S. Jarstad, MD, FAAO, FRSM UK(oph), Professor of Clinical Ophthalmology Comprehensive, Cataract & Refractive Surgery, Department of Ophthalmology, Tampa for his contribution in English language editing.

Conflict of interest

The author declares no conflict of interest.

Author details

Sharita Siregar[1,2]

1 Cornea, Cataract and Refractive Surgery Division, JEC Eye Hospitals, Central Jakarta, Indonesia

2 Lions Eye Bank Jakarta, West Jakarta, Indonesia

*Address all correspondence to: doktertasha@gmail.com

References

[1] Niederkorn JY. The immune privilege of corneal allografts. Transplantation. 1999;67(12):1503-1508.

[2] Streilein JW. New thoughts on the immunology of corneal transplantation. Eye (Lond). 2003;17(8):943-948.

[3] Eghtedari M, Kamalzadeh M, Yasemi M, Movahedan H, Ashraf MJ. Five Years Pathological Evaluation of Corneal Regrafts: A Study from Southern Iran. J Ophthalmol. 2020; 2020:2546923.

[4] Guilbert E, Bullet J, Sandali O, Basli E, Laroche L, Borderie VM. Long-term rejection incidence and reversibility after penetrating and lamellar keratoplasty. Am J Ophthalmol. 2013;155(3):560-569 e2.

[5] Fasolo A, Capuzzo C, Fornea M, Franch A, Birattari F, Carito G, et al. Risk factors for graft failure after penetrating keratoplasty: 5-year follow-up from the corneal transplant epidemiological study. Cornea. 2011;30(12):1328-1335.

[6] Tuppin P, Poinard C, Loty B, Delbosc B. Risk factors for corneal regraft in patients on the French waiting list. Cornea. 2004;23(7): 704-711.

[7] Bell KD, Campbell RJ, Bourne WM. Pathology of late endothelial failure: late endothelial failure of penetrating keratoplasty: study with light and electron microscopy. Cornea. 2000; 19(1):40-46.

[8] Schaumberg DA, Dana R, Buring JE, Sullivan DA. Prevalence of dry eye disease among US men: estimates from the Physicians' Health Studies. Arch Ophthalmol. 2009;127(6):763-768.

[9] Schaumberg DA, Sullivan DA, Buring JE, Dana MR. Prevalence of dry eye syndrome among US women. Am J Ophthalmol. 2003;136(2):318-326.

[10] Barabino S, Chen Y, Chauhan S, Dana R. Ocular surface immunity: homeostatic mechanisms and their disruption in dry eye disease. Prog Retin Eye Res. 2012;31(3):271-285.

[11] Inomata T, Hua J, Nakao T, Shiang T, Chiang H, Amouzegar A, et al. Corneal Tissue from Dry Eye Donors Leads to Enhanced Graft Rejection. Cornea. 2018;37(1):95-101.

[12] Rayner SA, King WJ, Comer RM, Isaacs JD, Hale G, George AJ, et al. Local bioactive tumour necrosis factor (TNF) in corneal allotransplantation. Clin Exp Immunol. 2000;122(1):109-116.

[13] Dana MR, Qian Y, Hamrah P. Twenty-five-year panorama of corneal immunology: emerging concepts in the immunopathogenesis of microbial keratitis, peripheral ulcerative keratitis, and corneal transplant rejection. Cornea. 2000;19(5):625-643.

[14] Yamagami S, Dana MR, Tsuru T. Draining lymph nodes play an essential role in alloimmunity generated in response to high-risk corneal transplantation. Cornea. 2002;21(4):405-409.

[15] Boisgerault F, Liu Y, Anosova N, Ehrlich E, Dana MR, Benichou G. Role of CD4+ and CD8+ T cells in allorecognition: lessons from corneal transplantation. J Immunol. 2001;167(4):1891-1899.

[16] Yin XT, Zobell S, Jarosz JG, Stuart PM. Anti-IL-17 therapy restricts and reverses late-term corneal allorejection. J Immunol. 2015;194(8):4029-4038.

[17] Chen Y, Chauhan SK, Lee HS, Saban DR, Dana R. Chronic dry eye

disease is principally mediated by effector memory Th17 cells. Mucosal Immunol. 2014;7(1):38-45.

[18] Sagoo P, Lombardi G, Lechler RI. Relevance of regulatory T cell promotion of donor-specific tolerance in solid organ transplantation. Front Immunol. 2012; 3:184.

[19] Pflugfelder SC, Stern M, Zhang S, Shojaei A. LFA-1/ICAM-1 Interaction as a Therapeutic Target in Dry Eye Disease. J Ocul Pharmacol Ther. 2017;33(1):5-12.

[20] Perez VL, Pflugfelder SC, Zhang S, Shojaei A, Haque R. Lifitegrast, a Novel Integrin Antagonist for Treatment of Dry Eye Disease. Ocul Surf. 2016;14(2):207-215.

[21] Spurr-Michaud S, Argueso P, Gipson I. Assay of mucins in human tear fluid. Exp Eye Res. 2007;84(5):939-950.

[22] Lam H, Bleiden L, de Paiva CS, Farley W, Stern ME, Pflugfelder SC. Tear cytokine profiles in dysfunctional tear syndrome. Am J Ophthalmol. 2009;147(2):198-205 e1.

[23] Jensen OL, Gluud BS, Birgens HS. The concentration of lactoferrin in tears of normals and of diabetics. Acta Ophthalmol (Copenh). 1986;64(1): 83-87.

[24] Vinding T, Eriksen JS, Nielsen NV. The concentration of lysozyme and secretory IgA in tears from healthy persons with and without contact lens use. Acta Ophthalmol (Copenh). 1987;65(1):23-26.

[25] Zhou L, Huang LQ, Beuerman RW, Grigg ME, Li SF, Chew FT, et al. Proteomic analysis of human tears: defensin expression after ocular surface surgery. J Proteome Res. 2004;3(3): 410-416.

[26] De Paiva CS, Corrales RM, Villarreal AL, Farley WJ, Li DQ, Stern ME, et al. Corticosteroid and doxycycline suppress MMP-9 and inflammatory cytokine expression, MAPK activation in the corneal epithelium in experimental dry eye. Exp Eye Res. 2006;83(3):526-535.

[27] Simmons KT, Xiao Y, Pflugfelder SC, de Paiva CS. Inflammatory Response to Lipopolysaccharide on the Ocular Surface in a Murine Dry Eye Model. Invest Ophthalmol Vis Sci. 2016;57(6):2443-2451.

[28] Enriquez-de-Salamanca A, Castellanos E, Stern ME, Fernandez I, Carreno E, Garcia-Vazquez C, et al. Tear cytokine and chemokine analysis and clinical correlations in evaporative-type dry eye disease. Mol Vis. 2010; 16:862-873.

[29] Yoon KC, Jeong IY, Park YG, Yang SY. Interleukin-6 and tumor necrosis factor-alpha levels in tears of patients with dry eye syndrome. Cornea. 2007;26(4):431-437.

[30] Yoon KC, Park CS, You IC, Choi HJ, Lee KH, Im SK, et al. Expression of CXCL9, -10, -11, and CXCR3 in the tear film and ocular surface of patients with dry eye syndrome. Invest Ophthalmol Vis Sci. 2010;51(2):643-650.

[31] Choi W, Li Z, Oh HJ, Im SK, Lee SH, Park SH, et al. Expression of CCR5 and its ligands CCL3, -4, and -5 in the tear film and ocular surface of patients with dry eye disease. Curr Eye Res. 2012;37(1):12-17.

[32] Carreno E, Enriquez-de-Salamanca A, Teson M, Garcia-Vazquez C, Stern ME, Whitcup SM, et al. Cytokine and chemokine levels in tears from healthy subjects. Acta Ophthalmol. 2010;88(7): e250-e258.

[33] Zlotnick A, Mitchell RS, Brenner SL. recA protein filaments bind two

molecules of single-stranded DNA with off rates regulated by nucleotide cofactor. J Biol Chem. 1990;265(28): 17050-17054.

[34] Brignole F, Pisella PJ, Goldschild M, De Saint Jean M, Goguel A, Baudouin C. Flow cytometric analysis of inflammatory markers in conjunctival epithelial cells of patients with dry eyes. Invest Ophthalmol Vis Sci. 2000;41(6): 1356-1363.

[35] Springer TA. Adhesion receptors of the immune system. Nature. 1990;346(6283):425-434.

[36] Schaumburg CS, Siemasko KF, De Paiva CS, Wheeler LA, Niederkorn JY, Pflugfelder SC, et al. Ocular surface APCs are necessary for autoreactive T cell-mediated experimental autoimmune lacrimal keratoconjunctivitis. J Immunol. 2011;187(7):3653-3662.

[37] Stern ME, Schaumburg CS, Siemasko KF, Gao J, Wheeler LA, Grupe DA, et al. Autoantibodies contribute to the immunopathogenesis of experimental dry eye disease. Invest Ophthalmol Vis Sci. 2012;53(4): 2062-2075.

[38] Stern ME, Gao J, Schwalb TA, Ngo M, Tieu DD, Chan CC, et al. Conjunctival T-cell subpopulations in Sjogren's and non-Sjogren's patients with dry eye. Invest Ophthalmol Vis Sci. 2002;43(8):2609-2614.

[39] Yamagami S, Kawashima H, Tsuru T, Yamagami H, Kayagaki N, Yagita H, et al. Role of Fas-Fas ligand interactions in the immune rejection of allogeneic mouse corneal transplants. Transplantation. 1997;64(8):1107-1111.

[40] Stuart PM, Griffith TS, Usui N, Pepose J, Yu X, Ferguson TA. CD95 ligand (FasL)-induced apoptosis is necessary for corneal allograft survival. J Clin Invest. 1997;99(3):396-402.

[41] Liechtenstein T, Dufait I, Bricogne C, Lanna A, Pen J, Breckpot K, et al. PD-L1/PD-1 Co-Stimulation, a Brake for T cell Activation and a T cell Differentiation Signal. J Clin Cell Immunol. 2012; S12.

[42] Shen L, Jin Y, Freeman GJ, Sharpe AH, Dana MR. The function of donor versus recipient programmed death-ligand 1 in corneal allograft survival. J Immunol. 2007;179(6): 3672-3679.

[43] Yang W, Li H, Chen PW, Alizadeh H, He Y, Hogan RN, et al. PD-L1 expression on human ocular cells and its possible role in regulating immune-mediated ocular inflammation. Invest Ophthalmol Vis Sci. 2009;50(1):273-280.

[44] Chong EM, Dana MR. Graft failure IV. Immunologic mechanisms of corneal transplant rejection. Int Ophthalmol. 2008;28(3):209-222.

[45] Jiang L, He H, Yang P, Lin X, Zhou H, Huang X, et al. Splenic CD8+ T cells secrete TGF-beta1 to exert suppression in mice with anterior chamber-associated immune deviation. Graefes Arch Clin Exp Ophthalmol. 2009;247(1):87-92.

[46] Stein-Streilein J, Streilein JW. Anterior chamber associated immune deviation (ACAID): regulation, biological relevance, and implications for therapy. Int Rev Immunol. 2002;21(2-3):123-152.

[47] Wilbanks GA, Streilein JW. Studies on the induction of anterior chamber-associated immune deviation (ACAID). 1. Evidence that an antigen-specific, ACAID-inducing, cell-associated signal exists in the peripheral blood. J Immunol. 1991;146(8):2610-2617.

[48] Streilein JW. Anterior chamber associated immune deviation: the

privilege of immunity in the eye. Surv Ophthalmol. 1990;35(1):67-73.

[49] Yao YF, Inoue Y, Miyazaki D, Hara Y, Shimomura Y, Tano Y, et al. Correlation of anterior chamber-associated immune deviation with suppression of corneal epithelial rejection in mice. Invest Ophthalmol Vis Sci. 1997;38(2):292-300.

[50] Complete sequence and gene map of a human major histocompatibility complex. The MHC sequencing consortium. Nature. 1999;401(6756): 921-3.

[51] Streilein JW. Immunobiology and immunopathology of corneal transplantation. Chem Immunol. 1999; 73:186-206.

[52] Niederkorn JY. Mechanisms of corneal graft rejection: the sixth annual Thygeson Lecture, presented at the Ocular Microbiology and Immunology Group meeting, October 21, 2000. Cornea. 2001;20(7):675-679.

[53] Hamrah P, Zhang Q, Liu Y, Dana MR. Novel characterization of MHC class II-negative population of resident corneal Langerhans cell- type dendritic cells. Invest Ophthalmol Vis Sci. 2002;43(3):639-646.

[54] Stern ME, Gao J, Siemasko KF, Beuerman RW, Pflugfelder SC. The role of the lacrimal functional unit in the pathophysiology of dry eye. Exp Eye Res. 2004;78(3):409-416.

[55] Zhang MC, Liu X, Jin Y, Jiang DL, Wei XS, Xie HT. Lamellar keratoplasty treatment of fungal corneal ulcers with acellular porcine corneal stroma. Am J Transplant. 2015;15(4):1068-1075.

[56] Thygesen J, Aaen K, Theodorsen F, Kessing SV, Prause JU. Short-term effect of latanoprost and timolol eye drops on tear fluid and the ocular surface in patients with primary open-angle glaucoma and ocular hypertension. Acta Ophthalmol Scand. 2000;78(1):37-44.

[57] Mocan MC, Uzunosmanoglu E, Kocabeyoglu S, Karakaya J, Irkec M. The Association of Chronic Topical Prostaglandin Analog Use with Meibomian Gland Dysfunction. J Glaucoma. 2016;25(9):770-774.

[58] Osborne SA, Montgomery DM, Morris D, McKay IC. Alphagan allergy may increase the propensity for multiple eye-drop allergy. Eye (Lond). 2005;19(2):129-137.

[59] Sherwood MB, Grierson I, Millar L, Hitchings RA. Long-term morphologic effects of antiglaucoma drugs on the conjunctiva and Tenon's capsule in glaucomatous patients. Ophthalmology. 1989;96(3):327-335.

[60] Baudouin C, Liang H, Hamard P, Riancho L, Creuzot-Garcher C, Warnet JM, et al. The ocular surface of glaucoma patients treated over the long term expresses inflammatory markers related to both T-helper 1 and T-helper 2 pathways. Ophthalmology. 2008; 115(1):109-115.

[61] Baudouin C, Garcher C, Haouat N, Bron A, Gastaud P. Expression of inflammatory membrane markers by conjunctival cells in chronically treated patients with glaucoma. Ophthalmology. 1994;101(3):454-460.

[62] Baudouin C, de Lunardo C. Short-term comparative study of topical 2% carteolol with and without benzalkonium chloride in healthy volunteers. Br J Ophthalmol. 1998;82(1):39-42.

[63] Albietz JM, Lenton LM, McLennan SG. Chronic dry eye and regression after laser in situ keratomileusis for myopia. J Cataract Refract Surg. 2004;30(3):675-684.

[64] Belmonte C, Acosta MC, Gallar J. Neural basis of sensation in intact and injured corneas. Exp Eye Res. 2004;78(3):513-525.

[65] Sloniecka M, Le Roux S, Zhou Q, Danielson P. Substance P Enhances Keratocyte Migration and Neutrophil Recruitment through Interleukin-8. Mol Pharmacol. 2016;89(2):215-225.

[66] Kuchle M, Cursiefen C, Nguyen NX, Langenbucher A, Seitz B, Wenkel H, et al. Risk factors for corneal allograft rejection: intermediate results of a prospective normal risk keratoplasty study. Graefes Arch Clin Exp Ophthalmol. 2002;240(7):580-584.

[67] Calonge M. The treatment of dry eye. Surv Ophthalmol. 2001;45 Suppl 2: S227-S239.

[68] Aragona P, Papa V, Micali A, Santocono M, Milazzo G. Long term treatment with sodium hyaluronate-containing artificial tears reduces ocular surface damage in patients with dry eye. Br J Ophthalmol. 2002;86(2):181-184.

[69] Alldredge OC, Krachmer JH. Clinical types of corneal transplant rejection. Their manifestations, frequency, preoperative correlates, and treatment. Arch Ophthalmol. 1981;99(4):599-604.

[70] Claerhout I, Beele H, De Bacquer D, Kestelyn P. Factors influencing the decline in endothelial cell density after corneal allograft rejection. Invest Ophthalmol Vis Sci. 2003;44(11): 4747-4752.

[71] Hill JC, Maske R, Watson P. Corticosteroids in corneal graft rejection. Oral versus single pulse therapy. Ophthalmology. 1991;98(3):329-333.

[72] Batchelor JR, Casey TA, Werb A, Gibbs DC, Prasad SS, Lloyd DF, et al. HLA matching and corneal grafting. Lancet. 1976;1(7959):551-554.

[73] Roelen DL, van Beelen E, van Bree SP, van Rood JJ, Volker-Dieben HJ, Claas FH. The presence of activated donor HLA class I-reactive T lymphocytes is associated with rejection of corneal grafts. Transplantation. 1995;59(7):1039-1042.

[74] Volker-Dieben HJ, Schreuder GM, Claas FH, Doxiadis, II, Schipper RF, Pels E, et al. Histocompatibility and corneal transplantation. Dev Ophthalmol. 2003; 36:22-41.

[75] Reinhard T, Bohringer D, Enczmann J, Kogler G, Mayweg S, Wernet P, et al. Improvement of graft prognosis in penetrating normal risk keratoplasty by HLA class I and II matching. Eye (Lond). 2004;18(3): 269-277.

[76] Beekhuis WH, Bartels M, Doxiadis, II, van Rij G. Degree of compatibility for HLA-A and -B affects outcome in high-risk corneal transplantation. Dev Ophthalmol. 2003; 36:12-21.

[77] The collaborative corneal transplantation studies (CCTS). Effectiveness of histocompatibility matching in high-risk corneal transplantation. The Collaborative Corneal Transplantation Studies Research Group. Arch Ophthalmol. 1992;110(10):1392-1403.

[78] Treseler PA, Foulks GN, Sanfilippo F. Expression of ABO blood group, hematopoietic, and other cell-specific antigens by cells in the human cornea. Cornea. 1985;4(3): 157-168.

[79] Sano Y, Ksander BR, Streilein JW. Minor H, rather than MHC, alloantigens offer the greater barrier to successful orthotopic corneal transplantation in mice. Transpl Immunol. 1996;4(1): 53-56.

Chapter 7

Intense Pulse Laser Therapy and Dry Eye Disease

Sana Niazi and Farideh Doroodgar

Abstract

The high and increasing prevalence of Dry Eye Disease (DED) highlights the need for new treatment treatments and more effective management strategies for this chronic disease. After training, lid grooming, and various ocular lubricants, the Tear Film & Ocular Surface Society Dry Eye Workshop II (TFOS DEWS II) Management and Therapy Subcommittee recently proposed Intense Pulsed Light (IPL) as the second phase of therapy. Brief flashes of non-coherent light (400–1,200 nm) are delivered to the skin's surface using IPL technology. Toyos et al. found in 2005 that rosacea sufferers who were treated with IPL in the periocular region had a significant increase in their dry eye symptoms.

Keywords: intense pulse laser, dry eye disease, meibomian gland, MGD

1. Introduction

The lipid layer of the tear film is deficient when the activity of the meibomian glands is impaired, which protects the aqueous layer of the tear film and prevents it from evaporating. The cornea is exposed as the tear film is destabilized, which leads to the onset of DED symptoms [1]. Since facial rosacea is closely linked to Meibomian Gland Dysfunction (MGD) and blepharitis [1], the IPL intervention of rosacea may have removed pathological telangiectasia periocular area, eliminating a significant source of inflammation to the eyelids and, as a result, alleviating MGD and dry eye problems. Since Toyos' original publication, a slew of surveys and two Randomized Controlled Trials (RCT) [1, 2] have added to the body of evidence demonstrating the effectiveness (and safety) of IPL therapy for patients with DED caused by MGD [3]. Most of these studies showed that symptoms and a wide range of DED/MGD signals enhanced in these patients, such as Tear Breakup Time (TBUT), Non-Invasive Breakup Time (NIBUT), Schirmer examination, presence of phEx™. Tear inflammatory markers, lipid layer grade, lipid layer thickness, Corneal Fluorescein Staining (CFS), meibum consistency, meibum expressibility, and lid margin anomalies were investigated.

2. Definition and history of DED

Dry Eye Syndrome or Disease (DES or DED) is a chronic Ocular Surface Disease (OSD) that influences vision and, consequently, quality of life similar to angina pectoris.

The prevalence of DE varies by region and population, ranging from 5–50% and up to 75%. Female gender, Age, excessive cold or hot weather, low relative humidity,

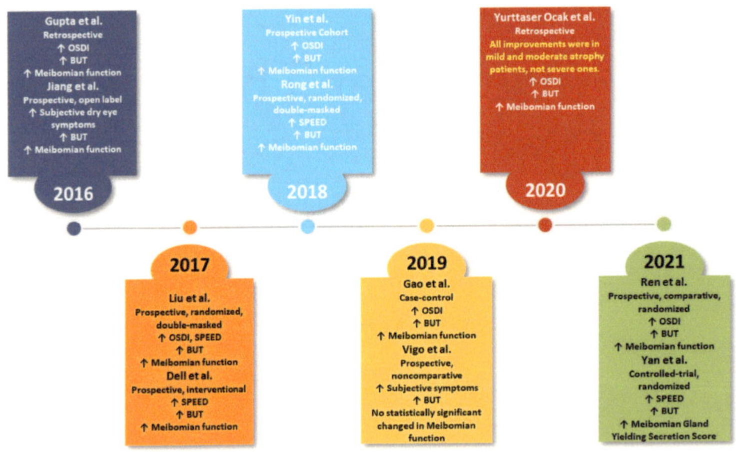

Figure 1.
Timeline diagram: IPL for DED treatment; ↑: Improvement, OSDI: Ocular surface disease index, BUT: Break up time, SPEED: Standard patient evaluation of eye dryness questionnaire.

proximity to video monitor terminals, contact lens wear, history of refractive surgery, smoking, and prescriptions are some risk factors [4–13].

Geographical area, research demographic differences, and a lack of consistent diagnosis criteria are thought to cause the significant disparity of prevalence worldwide (**Figure 1**) [13].

3. Diagnose of DED

There is not a gold standard for diagnosing dry eye disease. However, evaluations can arise from the following methods:

3.1 Standard patient evaluation of eye dryness (SPEED) questionnaire

This validated questionnaire [1, 14] asked the subject to grade the frequency and severity of four symptoms categories: (1) dryness, grittiness, or scratchiness; (2) soreness or irritation; (3) burning or watering; and (4) eye fatigue. For each of these symptom categories, the subject subs-cored the frequency using a 4-point scale (0 = never, 1 = sometimes, 2 = often, 3 = constant), and sub-scored the severity using a 5-point scale (0 = none, 1 = tolerable, 2 = uncomfortable, 3 = bothersome, 4 = intolerable). The SPEED score was calculated as the sum of these eight sub-scores. A SPEED score ≥ of 10 is widely accepted as indicating severe DED symptoms, 12. A cut-off value around six is often used to distinguish between asymptomatic/mild and moderate/severe symptoms.

3.2 Corneal fluorescein staining (CFS)

Assessment of corneal staining was evaluated as follow: [15]. Immediately following TBUT measurement and taking advantage of the residual staining in the ocular surface, the examiner observed four anatomical quadrants of the cornea (temporal superior, temporal inferior, nasal superior, nasal inferior) under the slit-lamp. Each quadrant was sub-scored using a 4-point scale; 0: no staining, 1: 1–30 instances of punctate staining, 2: 30 instances of punctate staining, without infused lesions or ulcers, or 3: the existence of infused lesions or ulcers. The sum of these four sub-scores, ranging from 0 to 12, defined the CFS score. The CFS score was evaluated at baseline (BL) and follow-up (FU).

3.3 Composite eyelid score (CES) and change of compound eyelid score (CCES)

A Composite Eyelid Score (CES) was compounded based on the presence or absence of five abnormal anatomical features of the eyelids: (1) hyperemia of anterior lid margin; (2) thicken lid margin; (3) rounded lid margin; (4) hyper-keratinization of the lid margin; and (5) telangiectasia around meibomian gland orifices.

These five features were evaluated at BL and FU. Each one was sub-scored 1 if the abnormality was present, or 0 otherwise. In the analysis, CES was calculated as the sum of these five sub-scores, thus ranging from 0 (all five features absent) to 5 (all five features present). At FU, the examiner used photos of the eyelids captured at BL to determine whether there was an improvement (+1), no change (0), or a deterioration (21) for each of these features. The sum of these five sub-scores, ranging from 25 (if all five features deteriorated) to +5 (if all five features improved), was defined as the Change in CES (CCES).

3.4 Tear breakup time (TBUT)

The diagnosis subcommittee on the International Workshop on MGD proposed that TBUT ranges of 1 to 3 sec, 3 to 5 sec, and 5 to 7 sec indicate moderate, mild, and minimal severity levels, respectively.

3.5 Ocular surface disease index (OSDI)

OSDI (Allergan, Inc., Irvine, CA) is a frequently used instrument to assess DE and provides a quantifiable assessment of DE symptom frequency and the impact of these symptoms on vision-related functioning. It contains 12 items, and the score can range from 0 (no symptoms) to 100 (severe symptoms) points; 0 to 12 represents normal, 13 to 22 represents mild DED, 23 to 32 represents moderate DED, and greater than 33 represents severe DED.

3.6 Tear film lipid layer (TFLL) quality by TFLL interferometry

Noninvasive TFLL quality assessment was performed with DR-1 (Kowa, Nagoya, Japan). Yokoi DE severity grading system was performed. Grade 1: somewhat gray color, uniform distribution; grade 2: rather gray color, nonuniform distribution; grade 3: a few colors, nonuniform distribution; grade 4: many colors, nonuniform distribution; and grade 5: corneal surface partially. 24 of refractive, refractive.

3.7 Meibum gland (MG)

The quality of the meibum was assessed by expressing the meibomian glands with the Meibomian Gland Evaluator (MGE; Tear Science, Inc., Morrisville, NC), a standardized instrument developed by Korb et al., and then evaluating the quality of meibomian secretions [16]. MGE was applied for 15 glands (5 nasal+5 central+5 temporals) along the lower eyelid. For each gland, the examiner sub-scored the quality of the expressed meibum using a four-point scale: 0 (no secretion), 1 (inspissated or toothpaste-like secretion), 2 (cloudy liquid secretion), or 3 (clear liquid secretion). The sum of this 15 subs-cores, ranging from 0 to 45, defined the Meibomian Gland Yielding Secretion Score (MGYSS). MGYSS was evaluated at BL and FU [1].

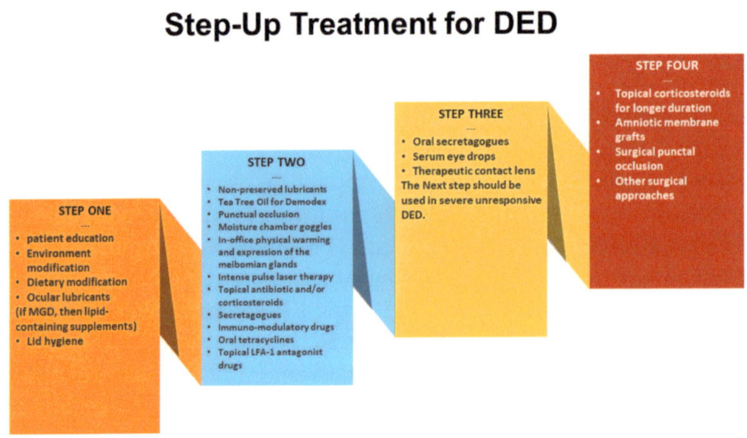

Figure 2.
Step-up treatment for DED.

4. Enhanced management and treatment for dry eye (DE)

The 2017 TFOS DEWS II provides guidelines for a stepped treatment protocol for DE, which targets each abnormality in the Tear Film-Oriented Diagnosis (TFOD) approach (**Figure 2**) [17–19].

4.1 Drug therapy

The inflammation, along with dry eye usually treats with topical corticosteroids. In cases with little satisfaction, a second-line drug is Topical cyclosporine A [20].

Lifitegrast 5% is a second topical anti-inflammatory ocular drop that got FDA approved In July 2016 for DED.

Other drugs include lipid-containing eye drop, artificial tear formulations with nanostructured lipid carriers as a synthetic TF in vivo, and castor oil emulsions are promising as Preservative-free drops, omega-3 fatty acid, supplementation, serum tears, topical azithromycin, oral and topical HA oral doxycycline, topical 3% Diquafosol and cholinergic.

4.2 Procedures

Intense pulse light, lacrimal plug, lid massage and probing and expression of MG, warm compresses or vectored thermal pulsation, and amniotic membrane biologic corneal bandage lens have evolved to improve the signs and symptoms of DE.

5. Definition of IPL

An intense pulsed light (IPL) system is a non-laser large source of light that produces a non-coherent light output of broad wavelength, usually in the range of 500 to 1200 nm, using a high-performance flashbulb. Many modern tools create light pulses by transmitting bursts of electricity running through a xenon gas-filled chamber [21–23].

The usage of IPL in medicine is based on the fact that unique load transfer targets (chromophores) can absorb photons from a wide range of light wavelengths (absorptive band) without being specifically targeted by their highest absorption.

The IPL uses targeted photo thermolysis, in which thermally induced radiation harm is restricted to the selected epidermis and dermis textured targets at the cellular or tissue structural difference [24]. Toyos et al. reported improvements in MGD associated Dry Eye Disease (DED) cases in 2002 and was the first published report on using an IPL system in ophthalmology [25, 26]. IPL dilates the capillaries and causes them to involute using electromagnetic waves of specific wavelengths [27]. This causes the leaked inflammatory responses to be suppressed, interrupting the vicious cycle of inflammation and enhancing dry eye signs. In most cases, it also functions with the aid of thermal pulsation [28]. When chronic inflammation occurs, the structure of the meibum improves to contain many monounsaturated fats. Those fats have a melting point of close to 45°C, which is greater than body temp [29]. This meibum does not melt through the lipid coating of the tear film as it should, clogging the glands. Thermal pulsation treatment liquefies the meibum and clears the glands by combining continuous pressure and heat. Traditional manual expressing glands is ineffective, inconvenient for patients, and could result in scarring [29]. Thermal pulsation is an effective and safe treatment option. With these processes in mind, we have deduced that IPL will help alleviate the symptoms of DE [21, 30].

6. Causes of dry eye and applications of IPL

The surface epithelial and glandular tissues (cornea, bulbar and palpebral conjunctiva, lacrimal and accessory eyelid), the glycocalyx, and the tear film consist of the microenvironment of the ocular surface [31].

Systemic disorders such as rheumatoid arthritis, Sjogren's syndrome, thyroid eye disease, sleep apnea [32], cicatrizing disease of the conjunctiva, contact lens wear, and refractive laser surgery are the most underlying associated conditions with Refractory DE. DE signs after Laser-Assisted in Situ Keratomileuses (LASIK) are not standardized. There is a continuum of disorders such as neurotrophic disease, tear film dysfunction, aqueous tear deficiency, and neuropathic pain conditions. Cutting the corneal nerves during Laser ablation and creating the flap are probable reasons for post-refractive DE. Meibomian glands are adjusted sebaceous glands located inside the lower and upper eyelids, with ducts terminating along the eyelid borders and secreting meibum, contributing directly to the lipid portion [31, 33].

The Tear Film Lipid Layer (TFLL) leads to the tear film's consistency and stabilization. The presence of TFLL on the tear film's exterior layer decreases the tear film's evaporation.

Negative TFLL changes may trigger evaporative DE, as well as symptomatic and clinical ocular surface manifestations [34]. Inflammation and illness TFLL were shown to be slightly lower in post-LASIK eyes, along with worsening DE symptoms and reduced corneal sensitivity [35].

A previous study reported the improvement of refractory DE with polar and nonpolar lipid base, ofloxacin eye ointment [36]. Another study reported the correlation between the severity of DE with lipid layer thickness secondary to increased evaporation as the most common etiologies for increased osmolarity of the tear film [37].

Scanning electron microscopy showed that lipids expressed by the meibomian gland caused extensive damage to gram-positive and gram-negative bacteria and hence acts as a protective barrier against pathogens [38]. Thus, improvement of the TFLL maintains the homeostatic balance by protecting the ocular surface environment. Therefore, the progress of symptoms and reduction of artificial tears after refractive surgery is another positive report about IPL treatment. However, future study elucidates the duration and the optimal dose [39, 40].

7. Mechanisms of IPL for prevention of damage to the ocular surface

A better explanation of the mechanisms of IPL leads to a better treatment plan. Regarding several mechanisms, it would be nice to describe as follow:

Demodex folliculorum and Bacillus oleronius are common inhabitants of human hair follicles and sebaceous glands occasionally found in ocular rosacea. IPL increases mitochondrial activity and wound healing, decreasing lid marginal bacteria and Demodex by photocoagulation, improving elastosis, and connective tissue disorganization that occurs with MGD rosacea to relieve pain (**Figure 3**).

7.1 Effects on mucin and corneal nerve

Mucin plays many essential roles on the ocular surface, including maintaining lacrimal fluid, lubricating the ocular surface to facilitate flat blinking, forming a smooth spherical surface for clear vision, providing an ocular surface shield and trapping and eliminating contaminants and debris [41–43]. The tear film is divided into two layers, with the aqueous layer containing secreted mucin MUC5AC scattered across [42]. Xue et al. discovered no improvements in MU5AC expression after IPL procedures Utilizing conjunctival impression cytology,. IPL therapy has little effect on the density of nerve fibers and dendritic cells in the corneal sub-basal layer, according to research [44].

7.2 Pro- and anti-inflammatory molecule effects, as well as matrix metalloproteinase suppression

Factors that influence tear film stability and osmolarity can cause ocular injury and trigger an inflammatory cascade that leads to a strong immunological reaction, leading to further ocular surface injury, causing a self-perpetuating inflammatory loop [45]. By upregulating anti-inflammatory cytokines, downregulating proinflammatory cytokines, or both, IPL can disrupt the inflammatory cycle. Dry eye's inflammatory cascade is highly complex and little known. Nevertheless, at least part of IPL's positive effect on DED patients may come from messing with the pathology's inflammatory cycle's positive feedback loop [46]. Interference with the inflammatory process by modulating anti-inflammatory factors and Matrix Metalloproteinase (MMP), lowering the turnover of skin epithelial cells, reducing the rate of severe obstruction of the meibomian glands, and improving the levels of active oxidative species all aid in the prevention of dry eye symptoms.

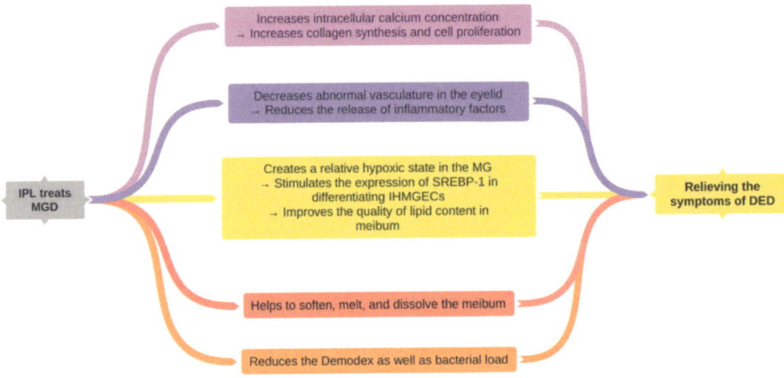

Figure 3.
IPL treats MGD; IHMGEC: Immortalized human MG epithelial cells; SREBP-1: Sterol regulatory element-binding protein 1.

8. Adverse events and advantages

There were no adverse effects with the IPL. Nevertheless, the relationship between Intense Pulsed Light (IPL) and Meibomian Gland Expression (MGX), or Warm Compresses (WC) and MGX, on the one hand, and MGX on the other hand, maybe non-linear and complex. Since IPL can be expensive in some clinics, it's essential to know if persistent eyelid warmth at home accompanied by WC/MGX can produce comparable results as IPL/MGX. However, Broadband Light (BBL) technology has the potential to cause damage. Just transient side changes were reported, such as hyperpigmentation, eyelash thinning, and slight conjunctival abrasion. The lid thinning has been seen by using higher settings than those prescribed in this report, and the suspected abrasion was most likely caused by slight damage caused by the corneal shields in the close eyelids' environment, rather than the BBL therapy itself. Other warnings that can help to reduce the low risk of transient lash thinning include scraping any gel that may couple with the light from the lashes and wrapping a metallic wrap around the edges of the cylinder to keep the treatment confined to the 7 mm circular adaptor's treatment area. To prevent any long-term risks, proper procedure and the use of correctly mounted, well-polished metallic eye shields are critical for corneal protection. It's important to remember that systems vary, and configurations can be tailored to the equipment in use and specific patient characteristics (skin texture, sun sensitivity, light-sensitizing drugs, and so on), with a thorough knowledge of the tissue effects at different settings/parameters [1].

8.1 IPL care has a risk vs. benefit ratio

Gupta et al. proved that IPL therapy for evaporative DED is a safe treatment in a study [47].

IPL appears to be a reliable and successful therapy for patients with evaporative DED, based on changes in quantitative clinical test results and subjective OSDI scoring evidence. The oil flow score and TBUT all increased significantly. There were no significant differences in intraocular pressure or acuity. There were no reports of ocular side effects. Some research found no adverse effects following IPL therapy and a substantial increase in MGD symptoms. In Chinese MGD cases with darker skin types (Fitzpatrick skin types III-IV), IPL treatment has also been effective and safe. Rong et al. found that strong pulsed light directly exposed to the eyelids, together with meibomian gland expression, effectively treats MGD [48].

IPL, in combination with MGX, was a safe and successful treatment for MGD. However, we must remember that the light beam emitted will be directed on a particular region, selectively damaging specific targets in the area being treated (e.g., capillaries, brown spots, or tattoo color in the skin), causing them to be eliminated or the region to be replaced with new cells—depending on the preferred procedure. IPL's effects can also be unwelcome, resulting in dangers like burns, blistering, and discomfort. Keloids and skin pigmentation are common severe symptoms. As a result, before proceeding with the procedure, the practitioner should advise the worried patients about the risks and benefits of IPL therapy. In meibomian gland dysfunction, intensive pulsed light therapy affects tear proteins, lipids, and inflammatory markers by controlling the amounts of total lipids, cholesterol, triglycerides, and phospholipids in the tear; IPL helps to alleviate the symptoms of DED. After IPL treatment, Ahmed et al. found substantial differences in tear protein concentrations and molecular weight [49]. The molecular weights of tear lysozyme, albumin, and lactoferrin were the most affected. The tears of MGD patients had slightly smaller levels of anionic phosphatidylethanolamine, phosphatidylserine, and phosphatidylinositol on thin-layer chromatography, however typical levels of zwitterionic neutral phospholipid phosphatidylcholine. After IPL treatment, these anionic phospholipids demonstrated impressive improvement. IPL enhances tear protein and lipid content and structure. Several studies have found IPL therapy reduces interleukin-6, interleukin-17A, and prostaglandin E2 levels in DED patients' tear fluid. Furthermore, they stated that a reduction in these inflammatory factors was related to decreased signs and symptoms. These decreases in inflammatory factors were linked to increases in corneal staining ratings, indicating that ocular surface epithelial damage had improved. According to some reports, changes in IL-6, IL-17A, and IL-1 levels were lowest one week after IPL, which was earlier than the appearance of clinical result peaks at one month. This means that increases in tear cytokine levels could be more sensitive indicators of IPL symptoms than clinical signs. IPL has an impact on the MGD meibum.

IPL has been shown in several trials to help release clogged meibum by thermal pulsation treatment. MGD is a critical contributor to dry eye illness with Sjogren disease, according to Godin et al. study's and should not be underestimated when evaluating care choices [50].

The meibum was able to clear its clogged ducts with the aid of thermal pulsation. Thermal pulsation is a treatment choice for patients with Sjogren's disease who have dry eye and MGD symptoms, and it will increase meibum consistency directly. Another research by yin et al. found that after therapy, TBUT, OSDI, MG expressibility, meibum quality, and MG dropout increased. IPL therapy significantly increased MG microstructure indices such as meibum, MG Acinar Unit Density (AUD), MG Acinar Longest Diameter (ALD), and the positive rate of Inflammatory Cells (ICs) across glandular structures. These results indicate that IPL therapy helps DED patients with MGD symptoms. It also increases eyelid hygiene and related ocular-surface indices, MG function, and MG macrostructure. Moreover, in MGD cases, IPL therapy primarily enhanced MG microstructure and reduces MG inflammation. MGD causes a difference in meibum content and quantity, which contributes to evaporative dry eye and ocular surface damage, increasing dry eye symptoms in certain people, according to Chhadva et al. on the meibum of MGD patients [51]. These modifications can be systemically managed with IPL, reducing the patient's difficulty [23, 31].

8.2 The advantages of IPL

Sufferers with refractory meibomian gland dysfunction are treated with intense pulsed light. Even more, research suggests that using strong pulsed light to treat MGD cases tends to alleviate dry eye symptoms. The aim of Arita et al. research.'s was to see whether strong pulsed light (IPL) combined with meibomian gland expression (MGX) could help with refractory meibomian gland dysfunction (MGD). Her findings indicated that combining IPL and MGX improved tear film homeostasis and alleviated ocular symptoms in cases with refractory MGD, making it a potential treatment option for this disorder. The meibomian gland activity was increased, the tear film was balanced, and ocular surface inflammation was reduced after IPL therapy. Meibum consistency, meibum expressibility, lid margin abnormality, ocular surface staining, tear film breakup period (TBUT), and the Ocular Surface Disease Index (OSDI) all improved significantly after IPL. Low meibum expressibility and a short TBUT were linked to a more significant improvement in the OSDI. Sufferers with refractory obstructive meibomian gland dysfunction responded well to IPL therapy combined with meibomian gland probing. Huang et al. discovered that, in comparison to IPL or Meibomian Gland Probing (MGP) alone, the mixture

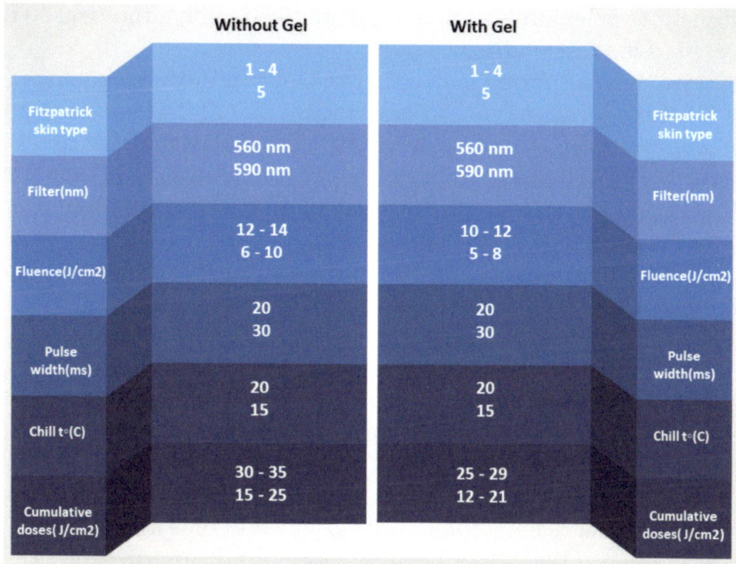

Figure 4.
Comparison of methods of IPL with and without gel.

MGP-IPL showed the most remarkable results in relieving all symptoms and signs and assisting patients in achieving long-term symptom relief [21, 52].

8.3 Evolution methods of IPL

The novel IPL/BBL from the high-intensity red (560–580 nm) to infrared (580–1200 nm) wavelengths of light may also improve blepharitis and DE by reducing Demodex and harmful bacteria [53]. This safe and effective protocol treats both the upper eyelid (more meibomian glands) and lower eyelids. It is now an off-label adaptation for ocular rosacea treatment (a form of MGD DED). Significant improvement of periocular symptomatology, MGD blepharitis symptoms, OSDI scores, and recurrence were observed with IPL/BBL after one year (**Figure 4**).

9. Discussion

Two types of IPL devices (E. Eye; E-SWIN, Paris, France, and Lumenis M22; Tel Aviv, Israel) were used in the studies. The E. Eye device produces a wavelength from 580 to 1200 nm, whereas the Lumenis M22 produces a 400 to 1200 nm wavelength. The broader wavelength of Lumenis M22 can theoretically achieve a better bactericidal effect. The light between 400 and 700 nm (415 most effectively absorbed) for *Propionibacterium acnes*, 500 nm, probably induces photo-thermolysis of vessels and prevents the leakage of inflammatory cytokines into the ocular surface. The yellow wavelength of IPL can target the oxyhemoglobin in superficial skin vessels, which have light absorption peaks of 578 nm. The sustained reduction in telangiectasia (decrease leakage of interleukins such as IL-17A and IL-6) was observed in patients with rosacea-related MGD after repeated IPL administration. On the contrary, the red-light spectrum (580–1200 nm) delivered by the E. Eye device has a more inadequate bactericidal effect. Still, it can potentially penetrate deeper into the skin and target the underlying sebaceous glands. And the use of the protective eye goggles is unclear or different between studies.

The different wavelength is another confounding factor, although 500 to 600 nm was used in most studies.

There are two intense pulsed light patterns: Optimal Pulse Technology (OPT) with three (3 weeks duration) consecutive treatments (10–14 J/cm^2) is more effective in improving MG function in lower eyelids and partial tear film signs than Intense Regulated Pulsed Light (IRPL) with four treatments (9–13 J/cm^2) on days (D)1, D15, D45, and D75 treatment. The method of light patterns used in each study causes a little disagreement.

Moreover, discrepancies between the ocular symptoms and signs of dry eye and the significant association of sleep disorders and ocular surface problems are common [54].

Besides, dry eye symptoms are more highly correlated with non-ocular conditions (sometimes somatization) than dry eye signs. The questionnaire does not any focus on a specific drug history for insomnia or antidepressants with anticholinergic effects.

It is also not irrational to conclude that identical findings would have been observed in a particular demographic with various skin type dispensation [23]. Another restriction was the lack of a gold standard for diagnosing and using TBUT as the essential result measure. Many reports of DED use tear breakup time; as a result, measure, but this outcome measure is troublesome for many reasons [23]. This procedure has a mild specificity/sensitivity. The findings are depending on the amount of coloring (fluorescein) ingrained in the eye, and the method is highly subjective to the observer's estimation. As a result, TBUT varies from one investigator to the next, even within the same investigator. While this averaging approach minimized TBUT measurement uncertainty, a more accurate and quantitative primary result indicator (e.g., NIBUT) may be a better option for investigation.

And finally, in the present pandemic, the eye route of infection must be considered so each sufferer should be treated as a potential coronavirus carrier. As a potentially beneficial method for treating and relieving the effects of DES and avoiding COVID-19, various compounds may be added into the food and then used as ready-made supplements. Polyunsaturated fatty acids had the most reported medicinal benefit, as they help alleviate the disease's infectious aspect. Vitamins, omega acids, and other nutritional nutrients can be discussed with each person individually.

10. Conclusion

To summarize, IPL is an attractive alternative solution for sufferers with DED caused by MGD, and that the effect of IPL is real rather than a placebo effect.

11. Take-home messages

It is essential to address the following points:

1. As we know, the MGD is not yet an approved indication for IPL therapy by the United States Food and Drug Administration. Regarding the safety of IPL and reported adverse events (14% of patients: cheek swelling, conjunctival cyst, floaters, blistering, hair loss at brow and forehead, light sensitivity, and facial redness). The IPL treatment should adhere to lower eyelids for now and in the presence of ocular protection due to the report about uveitis and iris damage. Although adverse effects usually resolved without treatment within one week

and iris damage has been reported during cosmetic IPL therapy on the upper eyelids by no ophthalmologic health care workers.

2. When we discuss about Intense Pulse Laser as a new treatment, confounding factors should be borne in mind: Age, baseline Ocular Surface Disease Index, MGD severity are potential factors that may influence the effects of IPL [55]. Some factors are difficult to control, such as patients' lifestyle, hormone levels, mood, and environment, which may affect the therapeutic effect of IPL treatment as follows:

    - Increased exercise and higher estrogen levels were also associated with improved tear quantity during the ovulation phase [56].

    - The majority of the available studies on nutritional supplementation [57] for DED did not evaluate the micronutrient dietary intake nor their plasma level, representing the major limitation of the existing literature. However, Epitropoulos et al., Malhotra et al., and Oleñik et al. showed significant improvement in OSDI, TBUT, lid margin inflammation, and meibum expressibility placebo, using Eicosapentaenoic Acid (EPA) + Docosahexaenoic Acid (DHA) [57].

    - On the other hand, sleep deprivation reduces androgen levels parasympathetic activity. It makes high levels of stress hormones (norepinephrine and cortisol) and reduce tear secretion lacrimal system function that reversed after 14 days of rest [58] (**Table 1**).

Abbreviations	Definitions
BBL	Broadband Light
BL	Baseline
BUT	Breakup Time
CCES	Change of Compound Eyelid Score
CES	Composite Eyelid Score
CFS	Corneal Fluorescein Staining
DE	Dry Eye
DED	Dry Eye Disease
DES	Dry Eye Syndrome
FU	Follow-up
ICs	Inflammatory Cells
IHMGEC	Immortalized Human MG Epithelial Cells
IPL	Intense Pulsed Light
IRPL	Intense Regulated Pulsed Light
LASIK	Laser-Assisted in Situ Keratomileuses
MG	Meibomian Gland
MG ALD	Meibomian Gland Acinar Longest Diameter
MG AUD	Meibomian Gland Acinar Unit Density
MGD	Meibomian Gland Dysfunction
MGE	Meibomian Gland Evaluator

Abbreviations	Definitions
MGP	Meibomian Gland Probing
MGX	Meibomian Gland Expression
MGYSS	Meibomian Gland Yielding Secretion Score
MMP	Matrix Metalloproteinase
NIBUT	Non-Invasive Breakup Time
OPT	Optimal Pulse Technology
OSD	Ocular Surface Disease
OSDI	Ocular Surface Disease Index
RCTs	Randomized Controlled Trials
SPEED	Standard Patient Evaluation of Eye Dryness Questionnaire
SREBP-1	Sterol Regulatory Element-Binding Protein 1
TBUT	Tear Breakup Time
TFLL	Tear Film Lipid Layer
TFOD	Tear Film-Oriented Diagnosis
TFOS DEWS II	Tear Film & Ocular Surface Society Dry Eye Workshop II
WC	Warm Compresses

Table 1.
Abbreviations and definitions.

Author details

Sana Niazi[1] and Farideh Doroodgar[2*]

1 Medical Students Research Committee, School of Medicine, Shahid Beheshti University of Medical Sciences, Tehran, Iran

2 Negah Specialty Ophthalmic Research Center, Shahid Beheshti University of Medical Sciences, Tehran, Iran

*Address all correspondence to: farinaz_144@yahoo.com

References

[1] Yan, X., et al., The efficacy of intense pulsed light combined with Meibomian gland expression for the treatment of dry eye disease due to Meibomian gland dysfunction: A Multicenter, randomized controlled trial. Eye and contact lens, 2021. 47(1): p. 45-53.

[2] Arita, R., et al., Multicenter study of intense pulsed light therapy for patients with refractory meibomian gland dysfunction. Cornea, 2018. 37(12): p. 1566.

[3] Toyos, R., C. Buffa, and S. Youngerman, Case Report: Dry-Eye Symptoms Improve with Intense Pulsed Light Treatment. Eye World News Magazine, 2005.

[4] Bakkar, M.M., et al., Epidemiology of symptoms of dry eye disease (DED) in Jordan: A cross-sectional non-clinical population-based study. Contact Lens and Anterior Eye, 2016. 39(3): p. 197-202.

[5] Hashemi, H., et al., Prevalence of dry eye syndrome in an adult population. Clinical and experimental ophthalmology, 2014. 42(3): p. 242-248.

[6] Lee, A., et al., Prevalence and risk factors associated with dry eye symptoms: A population based study in Indonesia. British Journal of Ophthalmology, 2002. 86(12): p. 1347-1351.

[7] Moss, S.E., R. Klein, and B.E. Klein, Prevalence of and risk factors for dry eye syndrome. Archives of ophthalmology, 2000. 118(9): p. 1264-1268.

[8] Onwubiko, S.N., et al., Dry eye disease: Prevalence, distribution and determinants in a hospital-based population. Contact Lens and Anterior Eye, 2014. 37(3): p. 157-161.

[9] Sendecka, M., A. Baryluk, and M. Polz-Dacewicz, Prevalence and risk factors of dry eye syndrome. Przeglad epidemiologiczny, 2004. 58(1): p. 227-233.

[10] Uchino, M., et al., Prevalence and risk factors of dry eye disease in Japan: Koumi study. Ophthalmology, 2011. 118(12): p. 2361-2367.

[11] Vehof, J., et al., Prevalence and risk factors of dry eye disease in a British female cohort. British Journal of Ophthalmology, 2014. 98(12): p. 1712-1717.

[12] Asbell, P., et al., Defining the needs and preferences of patients with dry eye disease. BMJ open ophthalmology, 2019. 4(1): p. e000315.

[13] Shanti, Y., et al., Prevalence and associated risk factors of dry eye disease in 16 northern west bank towns in Palestine: A cross-sectional study. BMC ophthalmology, 2020. 20(1): p. 1-8.

[14] Ngo, W., et al., Psychometric properties and validation of the standard patient evaluation of eye dryness questionnaire. Cornea, 2013. 32(9): p. 1204-1210.

[15] CDGoOS, C., Experts' consensus about clinical diagnosis and treatment of dry eye (2013). Chin Jophthalmol, 2013. 49: p. 73-75.

[16] Korb, D.R. and C.A. Blackie, Meibomian gland diagnostic expressibility: Correlation with dry eye symptoms and gland location. Cornea, 2008. 27(10): p. 1142-1147.

[17] Jones, L., et al., TFOS DEWS II management and therapy report. The Ocular Surface, 2017. 15(3): p. 575-628.

[18] Wolffsohn, J.S., et al., TFOS DEWS II diagnostic methodology report. The ocular surface, 2017. 15(3): p. 539-574.

[19] Hantera, M.M., trends in dry eye disease management worldwide. Clinical ophthalmology (Auckland, N.Z.), 2021. 15: p. 165-173.

[20] Buckley, R.J., Assessment and management of dry eye disease. Eye, 2018. 32(2): p. 200-203.

[21] Suwal, A., et al., Use of intense pulsed light to mitigate Meibomian gland dysfunction for dry eye disease. International journal of medical sciences, 2020. 17(10): p. 1385-1392.

[22] Raulin, C., B. Greve, and H. Grema, IPL technology: A review. Lasers in Surgery and Medicine: The Official Journal of the American Society for Laser Medicine and Surgery, 2003. 32(2): p. 78-87.

[23] Zhang-Nunes, S., et al., Safety and efficacy of an augmented intense pulse light protocol for dry eye syndrome and Blepharitis. Photobiomodulation, Photomedicine, and Laser Surgery, 2020. 39(3): p. 178-184.

[24] Anderson, R.R. and J.A. Parrish, Selective photothermolysis: Precise microsurgery by selective absorption of pulsed radiation. Science, 1983. 220(4596): p. 524-527.

[25] Toyos, R., W. McGill, and D. Briscoe, Intense pulsed light treatment for dry eye disease due to meibomian gland dysfunction; a 3-year retrospective study. Photomedicine and laser surgery, 2015. 33(1): p. 41-46.

[26] Song, W. and X. Yan, Research progress of intense pulsed light treatment on meibomian gland dysfunction and relevant dry eye diseases. [Zhonghua yan ke za zhi] Chinese journal of ophthalmology, 2018. 54(2): p. 140-143.

[27] Onesti, M. and P. Fioramonti, Intense Pulsed Light Systems, in International Textbook of Aesthetic Surgery. 2016, Springer. p. 1123-1131.

[28] Vegunta, S., D. Patel, and J.F. Shen, Combination therapy of intense pulsed light therapy and meibomian gland expression (IPL/MGX) can improve dry eye symptoms and meibomian gland function in patients with refractory dry eye: A retrospective analysis. Cornea, 2016. 35(3): p. 318-322.

[29] Macsai, M.S., The role of omega-3 dietary supplementation in blepharitis and meibomian gland dysfunction (an AOS thesis). Transactions of the American Ophthalmological Society, 2008. 106: p. 336.

[30] Sambhi, R.-D.S., et al., Intense pulsed light therapy with meibomian gland expression for dry eye disease. Canadian Journal of Ophthalmology, 2020.

[31] Pazo, E.E., et al., Intense pulse light for treating post-LASIK refractory dry eye. Photobiomodul Photomed Laser Surg, 2021. 39(3): p. 155-163.

[32] Bommert, C.M., et al., Sleep apnea and dry eye: How sleep apnea affects the eye surface. Ophtha Therapy, 2020. 7(2): p. 103-107.

[33] Greiner, J.V., Long-term (12-month) improvement in meibomian gland function and reduced dry eye symptoms with a single thermal pulsation treatment. Clinical and Experimental Ophthalmology, 2013. 41(6): p. 524-530.

[34] Blackie, C.A., et al., The relationship between dry eye symptoms and lipid layer thickness. Cornea, 2009. 28(7).

[35] Toda, I., Dry eye after LASIK. Investigative Ophthalmology and Visual Science, 2018. 59(14): p. DES109-DES115.

[36] Goto, E., et al., Successful Tear Lipid Layer Treatment for Refractory Dry Eye in Office Workers by Low-Dose Lipid Application on the Full-Length

Eyelid Margin. American Journal of Ophthalmology, 2006. 142(2): p. 264-270.e1.

[37] Foulks, G.N., The correlation between the tear film lipid layer and dry eye disease. Survey of Ophthalmology, 2007. 52(4): p. 369-374.

[38] Mudgil, P., Antimicrobial role of human Meibomian lipids at the ocular surface. Investigative Ophthalmology and Visual Science, 2014. 55(11): p. 7272-7277.

[39] O'Neil, E.C., et al., Advances in dry eye disease treatment. Current opinion in ophthalmology, 2019. 30(3): p. 166-178.

[40] Lam, P.Y., et al., A review on evidence-based treatments for Meibomian gland dysfunction. Eye and Contact Lens, 2020. 46(1): p. 3-16.

[41] Moniaux, N., et al., Structural organization and classification of the human mucin genes. Front Biosci, 2001. 6(1): p. D1192-DD206.

[42] Gipson, I.K. and P. Argueso, Role of mucins in the function of the corneal and conjunctival epithelia. Int Rev Cytol, 2003. 231(1): p. 1-49.

[43] Gipson, I.K., Y. Hori, and P. Argüeso, Character of ocular surface mucins and their alteration in dry eye disease. The ocular surface, 2004. 2(2): p. 131-148.

[44] Xue, A.L., et al., Randomised double-masked placebo-controlled trial of the cumulative treatment efficacy profile of intense pulsed light therapy for meibomian gland dysfunction. Ocul Surf, 2020. 18(2): p. 286-297.

[45] Yagci, A. and C. Gurdal, The role and treatment of inflammation in dry eye disease. International Ophthalmology, 2014. 34(6): p. 1291-1301.

[46] Dell, S.J., Intense pulsed light for evaporative dry eye disease. Clinical ophthalmology (Auckland, NZ), 2017. 11: p. 1167.

[47] Gupta, P.K., et al., Outcomes of intense pulsed light therapy for treatment of evaporative dry eye disease. Canadian Journal of Ophthalmology, 2016. 51(4): p. 249-253.

[48] Rong, B., et al., Intense pulsed light applied directly on eyelids combined with meibomian gland expression to treat meibomian gland dysfunction. Photomedicine and laser surgery, 2018. 36(6): p. 326-332.

[49] Ahmed, S.A., et al., Effect of intense pulsed light therapy on tear proteins and lipids in meibomian gland dysfunction. Journal of ophthalmic and vision research, 2019. 14(1): p. 3.

[50] Godin, M.R., S.S. Stinnett, and P.K. Gupta, Outcomes of thermal pulsation treatment for dry eye syndrome in patients with sjogren disease. Cornea, 2018. 37(9): p. 1155-1158.

[51] Chhadva, P., R. Goldhardt, and A. Galor, Meibomian gland disease: The role of gland dysfunction in dry eye disease. Ophthalmology, 2017. 124(11): p. S20-S26.

[52] Huang, X., et al., Clinic results of Intraductal Meibomian gland probing combined intense pulsed light in treating patients with refractory obstructive Meibomian gland dysfunction: A randomized controlled Trial. 2019.

[53] Cheng, S.-n., et al., Intense pulsed light therapy for patients with meibomian gland dysfunction and ocular demodex infestation. Current medical science, 2019. 39(5): p. 800-809.

[54] Lee, W., et al., The association between sleep duration and dry eye syndrome among Korean adults. Sleep Medicine, 2015. 16(11): p. 1327-1331.

[55] Chen, C., et al., Factors Influencing the Effectiveness of Intense Pulsed Light for Meibomian Gland Dysfunction. 2020, Research Square.

[56] Colorado, L.H., et al., Associations between the menstrual cycle, lifestyle factors and clinical assessment of the ocular surface: A prospective observational study. BMC women's health, 2020. 20(1): p. 23.

[57] Pellegrini, M., et al., The role of nutrition and nutritional supplements in ocular surface diseases. Nutrients, 2020. 12(4): p. 952.

[58] Monaco, G. and G. Casalino, Superficial keratectomy followed by intense pulsed light for Salzmann's nodular degeneration and coexisting meibomian gland dysfunction. European Journal of Ophthalmology, 2020: p. 1120672120964691.